PRAISE FOR *THIS IS SUPPOSED TO BE FUN*

"In a world full of one-size-fits-all sex and dating advice, *This Is Supposed to Be Fun* is a refreshing guide to understanding, celebrating, and challenging your unique needs and desires. Whether you're on all the apps or just looking to be in a sexier relationship with yourself, this book cuts through the complexity without ever flattening into stereotypes. It's a pleasure!"

—Ann Friedman, *New York Times*–bestselling coauthor of *Big Friendship*

"It's hard to stick out in the deluge of dating books that exist in the world promising to help you find 'the one,' but *This Is Supposed to Be Fun* does just that. Full of practical advice and prompts that encourage readers to get to the heart of their most authentic desires, this book is informative, realistic, and, most importantly, fun. *This Is Supposed to Be Fun* includes an in-depth analysis of how identity—especially race and gender—impacts your experience with dating, which is a welcome perspective shift given most accepted dating wisdom merely suggests the problem is you. I found myself not only enjoying the book but listing in my head all the friends I must send it to."

—Samhita Mukhopadhyay, former executive editor, *Teen Vogue*

"Myisha Battle brings deep compassion, true sex positivity, and respect for the role of pleasure-filled growth to the increasingly automated search for love and partnership. In this engaging and wonderfully written guide to dating and relationship-building, you'll find everything: a discussion of sexual values and compatibility, real talk about diversity issues and dating racism, and you'll learn how to extract the positive messages within rejection (and how to do no harm when you have to reject someone else). If you've regarded dating more as torment than as a personal-growth activity, you must pick up this book."

—Carol Queen, PhD, Good Vibrations Staff Sexologist

"*This Is Supposed to Be Fun* offers the first comprehensive, how-to guide for dating in the digital age, a time when the prospect of putting oneself out there can be daunting if not downright scary. Battle puts control back in the hands of daters, teaching them to think about what they want and how to get it, and how to become more connected to each other by first connecting deeply with themselves. There is no subject that goes unexamined, from flirting, to ghosting, and everything in between the sheets. This thoughtful, humane book reminds me, in a good way, of the sex-positive guides I snuck off my parents' shelves in the 1970s, but *This Is Supposed to Be Fun* addresses the sea change that has happened in the ensuing fifty years. Battle is an insightful voice of reason for those who feel lost in the wilderness of modern dating."

—Nancy Jo Sales, author of *Nothing Personal*

THIS IS
SUPPOSED
TO BE
FUN

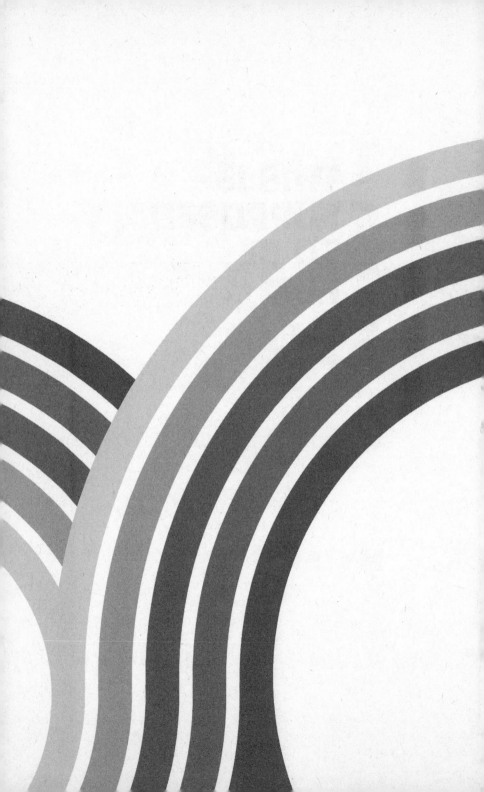

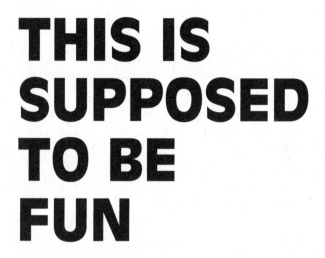

THIS IS SUPPOSED TO BE FUN

How to Find Joy in
Hooking Up, Settling Down,
and Everything in Between

MYISHA BATTLE

SEAL PRESS
NEW YORK

Seal Press
Hachette Book Group
1290 Avenue of the Americas, New York, NY 10104
www.sealpress.com
@sealpress

Printed in the United States of America

First Edition: January 2023

Published by Seal Press, an imprint of Perseus Books, LLC, a subsidiary of Hachette
Book Group, Inc. The Seal Press name and logo is a trademark of the Hachette Book
Group.

Names and identifying details have been changed. Characters are a composite.
Dialogue has been reconstructed from memory and compositely arranged. Any
similarity to actual persons is coincidental.

The Hachette Speakers Bureau provides a wide range of authors for speaking
events. To find out more, go to www.hachettespeakersbureau.com or email
HachetteSpeakers@hbgusa.com.

Seal Press books may be purchased in bulk for business, educational, or promotional
use. For information, please contact your local bookseller or Hachette Book Group
Special Markets Department at special.markets@hbgusa.com.

The publisher is not responsible for websites (or their content) that are not
owned by the publisher.

Print book interior design by Jeff Williams.

Library of Congress Cataloging-in-Publication Data

Names: Battle, Myisha, author.
Title: This is supposed to be fun : how to find joy in hooking up, settling down, and
    everything in between / Myisha Battle.
Description: First edition. | New York : Seal Press, 2023. | Includes bibliographical
    references.
Identifiers: LCCN 2022020439 | ISBN 9781541602212 (hardcover) |
    ISBN 9781541602137 (ebook)
Subjects: LCSH: Dating (Social customs) | Online dating.
Classification: LCC HQ801 .B3429 2023 | DDC 306.73—dc23/eng/20220518
LC record available at https://lccn.loc.gov/2022020439

ISBNs: 9781541602212 (hardcover), 9781541602137 (ebook)

LSC-C

Printing 1, 2022

Contents

PART 3:
LEAVE IT BETTER THAN YOU FOUND IT

Introduction

I thought this was supposed to be fun." The words hung heavy as my client Koya described the anxiety she was having about sorting through her matches on Bumble, a popular dating app. Everything felt so confusing and overwhelming. One minute she was chatting with a guy about pizza and the next he had unmatched her, disappearing completely from the chat. One guy asked for her number immediately after they had started chatting because he didn't want to check his messages on the app, and another was flooding her inbox with missives like "Good morning, beautiful," every single day, even though they hadn't met in person yet! This wasn't the first time she had attempted to date, but it had been years since she had invested herself in the process of trying to find a partner, or at the very least someone with whom she could have a stimulating conversation and hook up occasionally. And now she was second-guessing whether she should be trying at all.

As a sex and dating coach, I have worked with so many clients, like Koya, who are disillusioned with modern dating and unsure if they have the fortitude to get through all that is now required. The pervasiveness of app-based dating and the cultural shift away from meeting people organically in day-to-day life has set folks up for unique challenges when it comes to finding love, sex, and everything in between. If you're new to dating, figuring out where to start may seem daunting. And if this isn't your first time dating, you know that opting in means dealing with some flat-out fuckery, like ghosting, dead-end dates, and hooking up only to be let down by utterly unsatisfying sex. Maybe your experiences haven't been all bad; you just wish there was more of the good stuff, like connection, laughter, amazing sex, feeling seen and heard, and being truly on the same page with the people you're dating.

I can empathize with wherever you are in the process, because, like you, I had to commit to and navigate through what we now call dating to get what I wanted. I had dates that left me wondering, "What the fuck just happened?!" and I met some amazing people with whom I'm still in touch. I've been ghosted, stood up, slut-shamed, negged, misled, cheated on, emotionally played with, and generally disappointed. And I have to say, I've done my fair share of these things as well. But I've also fallen in love multiple times, learned about my sexuality, opened myself up to experiences and people I wouldn't have before, and confronted deeply held beliefs about what a "good relationship" looks and feels like for me.

From the very early days of my online dating journey, I felt alone. It seemed like everyone else was enjoying the ease of matching and going out on dates but me. I had questions about how gender, race, and class were playing out in my dating life, but I didn't have anyone to talk to about these things. I also believed at that time that any problem I was having finding what I wanted was my own, which made it even harder to pick myself up after an unpleasant experience.

When I decided to pursue a career as a coach, I knew I needed to integrate feminism and how cultural expectations impact dating into my coaching practice. My own dating experiences had shown me exactly how these expectations shaped most of the connections I made with people. Cultural misalignments regarding courtship, dating protocols, and sexual pleasure were everywhere—it wasn't just my perception. But back then I couldn't name it: the misogyny, the racism, the body and sex shame that were interwoven into my experiences as if they belonged there. And I surely didn't know what to do about it. I found myself and my needs taking a back seat to others', and I didn't know that I could demand more—from the process and from the people I was seeing.

It took a long time for me to figure out how to approach dating in a way that maximized the fun and minimized the bullshit. After years of conducting my own "field research" and building my private coaching practice where I guided others through the social minefields of dating, I'm now offering my insights to you. Because not only did I survive, but I also brought others with a wide array of identities, desires, and needs through to the other side of dating with more self-awareness, better connections, and (most importantly) more *fun* in their dating lives.

Each time I meet with a prospective client who wants help navigating the wild world of dating, I am thankful that I have enough experience in the trenches to serve as a realistic sounding board and guide for them. Knowing exactly what my clients go through has been the key to my success as a coach. If I didn't relate on a personal level to the good, the bad, and the utterly unbelievable bits of dating that my clients share with me, I honestly don't think I could do my job.

This book is meant to be your guide. I want the pages that follow to help you to move through the dating process, possibly multiple times, with a greater sense of ease. I know what it's like to feel like you're dating in a vacuum, with no one there who understands what's going on (sometimes including yourself). You might be the only one in your friend group who's single right now, or the pandemic may have lit a fire in you to start dating for the first time in a long time. You may have decided to open your relationship or start dating new types of people and you're not sure how to go about it. Regardless of how you're coming to this book and what your current dating goals are, I want to affirm your decision to figure it all out. And I don't want you to feel alone while you do it.

To that end, throughout the book I share the stories of my clients, who, like you, embarked on the brave work of forging their own path through dating. Each story is really an amalgam of experiences that clients have shared with me over the years and is meant to illustrate the most common concerns and scenarios that I've seen as a sex and dating coach. I take what my clients share with me seriously, and confidentiality is key to them feeling free to express what they need in our sessions. That's why I've changed names and identifying details and constructed composites to protect my clients' privacy. Scenarios and quotations have been reconstructed from memory and, in most cases, compositely arranged. Any similarity to actual persons is coincidental. I hope you can see yourself in these stories, take on the triumphs and lessons of my clients, and feel that much more empowered to move forward in your own dating life.

Though my work with each client is different, we always focus on a few key areas that, when addressed, provide more clarity and enjoyment throughout dating. That's why I've arranged the book in three helpful sections: Know Thyself, Do No Harm, and Leave It Better than You Found It. Each section is designed to address the stickiest parts of dating: knowing what the hell you want, creating great dates and sexual experiences, and either moving on from relationships that don't work for you or settling into the connections you've made.

Know Thyself will guide you through how you can clarify your goals before you even go on a date. I also provide my tried-and-true advice for how to attract great matches from the start so you can conserve your energy and avoid dating burnout. Do No Harm contains valuable strategies for setting up and going on dates, assessing compatibility throughout the dating process, and staying open (no matter how it's going). Leave It Better than You Found It encourages you to be compassionate when moving on from bad matches, breaking up, and giving feedback when there's a sexual misalignment. I'll also address how you can continue to grow within a new relationship.

In some ways, this book is a study of you. You'll have the opportunity to think about yourself and what you want from relationships in new ways. Throughout the book, I offer prompts and exercises to help you along your dating journey.

These will guide your focus inward to help you pinpoint the assumptions and habits that serve you, and the ones that don't. You may find it helpful to keep a journal handy as you read to take notes, respond to the prompts, and have something to refer back to as you're dating.

We all deserve to have fun on our romantic journeys, despite our differences. Who you are and the unique desires you hold should be celebrated, not hidden. I've watched my clients expand the amount of joy they have in dating as they boldly ask for and receive what they truly desire. I've seen them show up for themselves in new ways that attract different types of people and experiences, and I've seen matches move to dates to sex and relationships that enrich the lives of everyone involved. These folks, like you, started with an intention to make dating better for themselves. Whatever you're looking to improve in your dating life, I hope that by the end of this book you'll have the tools, language, and confidence necessary to go forth and create meaningful connections with people you actually like. It's that simple.

Now that I've outlined how I'd like you to use this book, here are a few things to keep in mind as you're reading:

1. Don't give up.
2. Try as much or as little as feels right for you at the time.
3. Stay open to possibilities.
4. Take what is useful and leave the rest.
5. Don't forget to take breaks when you need them.

With pleasure,
Myisha

PART 1
KNOW THYSELF

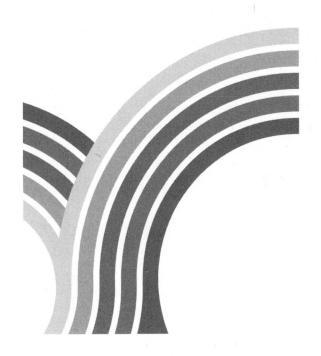

1

Who Are You and What the Hell Are You Doing Here?!

*If I didn't define myself for myself, I would be
crunched into other people's fantasies
for me and eaten alive.*

—AUDRE LORDE

Knowing who you are is hard work that literally takes a lifetime. Most of my coaching clients have done some work to understand who they are, but they have still found it challenging to hold on to their truths as they navigate relationships and sex. That's because most of us aren't encouraged to ask ourselves important questions about who we want to be as romantic partners and what relationship we want to have with sex throughout these partnerships. And what we want from relationships often depends on other areas of our lives—like career, health, and family—that change as we change. The kind of relationship we gravitate toward in our youth might not work with the demands of our later career goals. The need to be present for a sick parent or friend might alter the way we view what's important in a long-term partnership. Even learning more about what and who you like through the process of dating can dramatically shift what you believe you want when it comes to sex and partnership. It can be daunting to start the process of digging into who we are and prioritizing our sex and dating lives. But that's exactly what you're here to do—with me as your helpful guide, of course.

My hope is that by reading what I have to offer you in the chapters that follow and taking an active role in your own learning, you'll gain insight into yourself as you are now. This insight is the key to dating with confidence. The more you know yourself—why you believe what you do about the world and what you want from it—the more you'll be able to share that with others. And isn't that essentially what dating boils down to, sharing yourself with others and connecting with what they have to share with you?

You have a past that brought you to your current dating moment. You may understand and accept that past already, or you may need to unearth some buried history that, for better or worse, has been shaping your present dating life. Knowing where you come from and what messages you inherited about sex, dating, partnership, marriage, and family are the first steps to truly knowing who you are as a dater. When you meet prospective partners, you bring your ideas of how things *should* be into your dance of conversation and flirtation, and so do they. The thing is, most of us rarely question if what we're bringing to this dance is actually in our best interest. That's why it's such a good idea to do some introspection, to see if your expectations align with your current dating reality.

This chapter is all about exploring you. We'll dig into your past, bring to light how it may be impacting your current dating situation, and put these pieces together to form who you are as a dater right now. You're going to have lots of opportunities to explore your thoughts about dating, from what kind of relationships you ideally want to how masturbation fits into your dating life.

If you're excited, nervous, or a mix of both, that's okay! Take a moment to think about anything that is coming up for you now. It will be great to reflect back on these feelings later to see how you've changed.

KNOW YOUR HISTORY

How would you describe your upbringing in one sentence?

When forced to condense family history into a single thought, most people will comment on a few key factors that influenced how they were raised. It's common for folks to invoke descriptors of race, ethnicity, socioeconomic status or class, religion, and other cultural affiliations. These same descriptors can be used to examine how we developed our ideas about relationships, because our families are the proto-relationships we grow to understand and replicate.

You may have grown up with some pretty strong ideas about how romantic relationships work. You may have had religious or spiritual teachings that dictated when sexual contact could and couldn't happen, and you may have parents or close family members whose relationships seem to have followed along with these edicts. For you, it might feel like there is really only one path to relationship happiness.

Or, you may have rebelled against these ideals to pave your own way.

For those who grew up with examples of different types of relationship structures and expectations within your family, you may have seen so many ways to be in relationships that you internalized that making your own relationship rules was totally okay. You might sometimes feel overwhelmed by choices and unsure about which relationship structure could work for you. You may have even opted out of dating because there weren't any clear relationship success stories to hang on to on the bumpy path of your own dating life.

It's worth noting that many of us grew up with cisgender, heteronormative, monogamous examples of relationships that simply don't seem applicable to our own romantic and sexual development. This is especially true for LGBTQIA+ and polyamorous folks. The examples we get aren't always the ones we need.

Take Tasha, for instance. She was a client of mine who experienced major shifts in her thinking about her dating life when she started looking at her history. Each of my clients completes a sexual history and assessment before our first session together. Sometimes clients are eager to fill everything out and send in their responses. Others wait until the very last minute. Tasha was in the latter camp; she actually sent in her assessment minutes before her first appointment. I began that session by asking her what the process of reflecting on her sexual history was like for her, and she said it was more difficult than she thought it would be.

"I realize now that the thought of answering the questions in the assessment gave me a lot of anxiety, so I kept putting it off and putting it off. I knew I had to turn something in today so I just made myself do it. It was hard to reflect on how isolated I felt growing up. Being queer, I couldn't relate to any of my family. I was learning who I was attracted to, but I didn't have anyone to share that with. My sexuality felt dangerous, like something I had to protect other people from. Having to reflect on that, and think about how that impacts me now . . . It was really hard."

"Do you think that feeling of isolation has been impacting how you date as an adult?" I asked her.

"Maybe. I know so many people now who seem to have the life I want. They seem more confident in what they want and more adventurous when it comes to dating and hooking up. I tell my friends all the time how jealous I am that they seem to actually be having fun out there and I just feel stuck."

During the course of our work together, Tasha was able to create a vision for her future relationships based on a partnership model she believed was right for her. This model was inspired by what she found herself envying in her friends' relationships. She wanted commitment ultimately, but she also wanted fun and excitement and to feel like the people she was dating really saw and accepted her. This meant that she focused her search on people who were a little farther along in their own sexual and coming-out journeys, who could show her what was possible. By recognizing that she needed a different model from the one she had initially been given, she found the freedom and ability to seek out partners who helped her learn more and enjoy the process of dating.

Sometimes family provides just what we need. You may be someone who wants what your parents have, and that's great! I've had many clients whose major source of dating frustration was trying to find the kind of partnership that their parents or other important elders in their life have. We work together to make sure they are crystal clear about the relationship qualities they're looking to emulate, and then build these things into their dating profile and vetting process. You'll learn later on how to do this too!

There's no right or wrong when it comes to how we do our relationships. Whether or not you have a vivid picture of what you want your future relationship(s) to look like, just know that there are others out there like you who are trying to figure out who they are, find their person or people, and have a good time in the process.

GETTING PERSONAL

There's not a ton of space in life to think about the childhood messages we received about relationships, so I'm creating that space for you right here.

Let's start with a few questions about you.

- How did you feel about the relationships around you growing up? Did they seem like something to aspire to? Why or why not?

- Do you remember any messages about what a "good relationship" was? What were the key components?

- How would you describe your family's expectations of you and your relationships? For instance, do they encourage you to date or explore sexually, expect you to settle down, want grandkids immediately, etc.?

- How would you describe your relationship to relationships?

Now that you've thought through some of the ways that your upbringing has impacted how you feel about relationships, let's move on to how it might affect how you feel about sex.

NORMALIZING S-E-X

What messages about sex did you receive when you were growing up?

If you are like most people, you probably received conflicting messages that you're still trying to understand. Alongside the influence of our family, the culture we grow up in plays a big part in how we think and feel about sex. Every other pop song is about it, and we consume a ton of other media containing it, but just try talking about sex with other people (let alone a potential partner)! It can sometimes feel as if sex is simultaneously everywhere and nowhere at all. Like it's something we're supposed to want desperately but at the same time stress out about or even avoid. While most of us have a general belief that sex is a natural part of life, there's often much more to it than that.

Despite depictions of sexuality being everywhere, we actually live in a sex-negative culture. Despite our best efforts, we all have absorbed some form of sex negativity. The inability to feel comfortable voicing desires or talking openly about sex with people we trust points to a stigma that still exists: sex is to be *done*, not discussed. Yet the majority of my clients, whether single or partnered, list a lack of good sexual communication as one of the biggest obstacles in their relationships.

There is nothing inherently wrong or bad about having a sexual experience with someone (or many someones), but so often our culture reflects only the negative consequences of being sexual. This can lead to internalizing our desires and can create feelings of shame for wanting to be sexual, even when the conditions feel right for us. And if you identify as asexual, there is very little space in our culture to talk about what that might look like in relationships. There's an inherent sexualization to dating that might feel off-putting if that's not your main motivation for seeking connection. So whether sex is desired or not, you can be left feeling ashamed for wanting what you want.

If you are looking to have sex as a component of your dating experience, and you've never thought about what is right for you, here are a few common questions I am frequently asked to help you get started.

- Should you have sex on a first date?
- How many partners should you have before settling down?
- Can a relationship survive infidelity?
- What are the best sexual positions for maximum pleasure?
- Is it okay not to orgasm during sex?
- Should sexual compatibility be a prerequisite for partnership?

- Can you grow to become sexually attracted to someone you're not initially attracted to?

Chances are you have answers to some if not all of the above questions. But are these *your* answers? Are they conclusions you have come to because of your own experiences? Or are these answers you have absorbed from your upbringing or culture? Do these answers feel right for you now?

In my professional opinion, the answer to all of these questions is "It depends." So much of how we experience, process, and enjoy sexual relationships depends on what we *think* about sex. That's why, regardless of how you answered, there is a lot to learn about why you think the way you do about sex. You may know people who don't adhere to or reflect the answers you just provided. Do you have judgments of them? It's worth exploring how your beliefs differ from those of people around you and even, if it feels comfortable, talking openly with them about their beliefs and how they came to them. Sex often feels like an off-limits subject because we're not sure how other people feel about it, but that's actually a great place to start the conversation.

Knowing your own beliefs about sex and how you came to them can be extremely helpful in your search for partners. Having this knowledge will help you communicate yourself and your desires more effectively throughout the dating process. For instance, if you believe that having sex on a first date is not okay, and you are faced with the option to do so, it will be helpful for you to know why you believe this so you can make a decision based on what you need and desire in the moment.

TO HOOK UP OR NOT TO HOOK UP?

We all live with a tremendous amount of cultural pressure to keep things casual in dating. Millions of people use dating apps that have a reputation for facilitating easy hookups. The concept is so widespread, it sometimes feels like hooking up and dating are one and the same. They're not! Hooking up is a part of dating that you can choose to engage in or not.

If you have a strong belief that casual sex is wrong, then you may have resisted hookup culture. But if you're anything like my client Sierra, you may have dipped a toe or two into the hookup pool.

Sierra came to me looking for guidance through the wild world of online dating. A recent grad, she told me that she was ready to look for something serious. All throughout college, she had limited her relationships to a hookup here and there while she focused on her studies. She also had an extensive calendar of extracurriculars, so there just wasn't any time for more than the occasional sex sesh. She was okay with this as a means to a sexual end, but now she was ready for more, and it was proving difficult.

After moving cross-country for an amazing job opportunity, Sierra found herself in an unfamiliar situation: she no longer had a community of friends to introduce her to potential partners, and she was floundering between one-night stands and having to actually go on dates . . . sometimes in the light of day! Then she said something I hear time and time again: "I just don't know what to do, or what to say. This is all very new to me, and I just feel like I'm really bad at it."

Sierra, like so many of my clients, grew up hearing messages about her education being the most important thing, while romantic relationships were potential impediments to her success. It was just easier, and culturally expected, to keep relationships in the hookup zone. I have seen this across the gender spectrum and in folks who identify as all different orientations. Hooking up is often seen as a way to let off some sexual steam (and it definitely can be!), but folks who hook up exclusively can struggle with a lack of practical dating skills—skills that Sierra was realizing she desperately needed now.

In our work together, Sierra shared that she was raised by a single mom most of her life. Her stepdad, who married her mom when Sierra was in high school, was an amazing human. She loved seeing her mom in love. When she thought about what partnership meant to her when she was younger, it was hard to admit, but she didn't value it much. She saw that her mom was happy, for the most part, being single and taking care of her. It naturally became important for Sierra to create a life for herself that felt similarly independent. A lot of our work focused on whether those childhood feelings were still valid. Some of them were. She wanted to be self-sufficient and autonomous, but she also craved a partner with whom she could share her wins and losses.

"I'm not someone who *needs* a partner. I actually love doing things on my own. But at the end of a long week, it would be nice to have someone to spend time with who really knows me," she explained.

"And you haven't had that experience so far with dating?" I asked.

"Not yet! Every time I meet someone, it always seems to result in a one-night thing, or it's casual for a few months and then peters out. It's exhausting starting from scratch every few months."

The more we talked, the more it became clear that she wanted out of the hookup loop—it just wasn't delivering what she needed anymore. Though it had served her needs in the past, she was learning about who she was becoming and what she wanted in her future. We worked on refining how she could express what she wanted from dating in her profile, expanding her practical experience going on dates, and reflecting on whether the folks she was meeting aligned with these new desires.

At the opposite end of the spectrum, my client Keaton needed a gentle nudge *into* the hookup pool. While he had been in two major long-term relationships, he was beginning to wonder whether his gauge for good partnerships was a bit off. His relationships always fizzled out sexually. He described both exes as being "really great friends," but the chemistry had never been that strong to begin with.

His sexual history involved becoming intimate only when he was in a committed relationship, and he had often felt that he couldn't fully express himself sexually with his past partners. In truth, he didn't exactly know what he was looking for; he just knew that what he was doing wasn't working. He had recently been on a string of dates with women who expressed their sexual interest in him early on, and he had frozen on the spot. His tendency was to take his time, establish a friendship, and then move that relationship into sexual territory. He knew that hooking up was an option;

he just wasn't sure how he felt about it. Would it make him a bad person? Would he be taking advantage of someone? We talked about his upbringing and how sex was never really discussed except when mentioned in the context of marriage. He obviously wasn't waiting until marriage to have sex, but in the past he had experienced a lot of guilt when even considering a casual encounter. He realized that he had internalized the message that sex should only happen when there's some form of commitment.

After a while, Keaton was able to separate himself from the expectations of his family and realize that he was already on a different path. Why not push his boundaries a bit? One day, he began our session with "I did it!" and explained that he had had an amazing night with a woman who was passing through town for work. He was elated by his experience with her, stating that he had never felt that kind of intense sexual connection. They had hit it off on their first date, which became a twelve-hour-long dinner turned overnight experience.

"Are you feeling any guilt?" I asked.

"A little . . . but the pleasure of having such a strong sexual connection exceeds any guilty feelings. I've never connected with someone like that before. I always thought I was just more sexually reserved than everybody else, but I noticed myself letting go a bit more because I wasn't hung up on where this was going to go. The fact that she was leaving town meant that it was kind of now or never, and that was the push I needed to just go with the flow. I wasn't 100 percent sure we were going to have sex; I was just enjoying each moment."

"That's great! You learned what your sexual connection could be when you're less attached to the outcome of the relationship. That's huge! Think you'll do this again?"

Keaton paused. "I don't know, but I'm definitely more open to possibilities now!"

EXERCISE: CREATING A HOOKUP PROS AND CONS LIST

As with anything in life, you have to evaluate what you think is right when it comes to dating by weighing the pros and cons. What do you want to focus on right now? Gathering sexual experiences with no strings attached, connecting with other people who are interested in more, or both? There's no wrong answer, just arguments for and against based on what you feel will work best for you right now. Relationships can provide stability when they're with great matches, but feeling stuck with someone who drains your energy might be a huge setback. Hooking up to learn about yourself and what you like can be super fun, but what about when someone is a jerk or you find yourself wanting to keep things casual with someone who catches feelings for you?

I encourage you to create your own personal list of pros and cons for hooking up and relationships. Remember, this is an exercise for who you are now. Your past self may have thought differently, and you may look back on this in the future and think, "Wow! I've changed a lot." What matters is that you're getting to know how you feel about these types of situations as the person you are right now. Making a pros and cons list will allow you to tap into what makes sense for your life given your past experiences and your current beliefs and needs. That's how you start to build dating goals for the future!

THE GREATEST LOVE OF ALL

Now that you know how normal it can be to use dating as a way to learn about yourself and that hooking up is one of the many reasons people choose to date, it's time we talk about an often overlooked part of the dating process: masturbating. Why am I bringing masturbation up, and so soon? Because I frequently hear from my dating clients that they want to have healthy and fulfilling sex lives, but they never learned to self-pleasure and struggle with communicating what they like. Developing a masturbation practice is my primary recommendation to those clients who feel at a loss when it comes to knowing and describing what they want. Some of my clients are in partnerships with mismatched libidos, and they tell me that they masturbated more frequently when they were single. Now that they have a partner, they've thrown all their eggs into one sex basket—to disastrous effect. Masturbation is a great way for folks to take ownership of their own desires and balance the responsibility of satisfying those desires within a partnership. Whether you are single or partnered, masturbation can be a great outlet for expressing sexual desire. For these reasons, I encourage everyone to cultivate a masturbation practice that can be relied upon through thick and thin.

You are your first and longest-lasting sexual partner. Think about it: most of us start self-pleasuring at a very young age.

Your gender, culture, and upbringing will have influenced how you felt about it at the time, or even now, but the fact remains that, from early on, you do *you*! A lot of people think that masturbation is something to be ashamed of and grown out of, and that the goal of dating is to eradicate the need for this unseemly activity. This just isn't the case. Another person isn't responsible for fulfilling all of your sexual needs. And they shouldn't be asked to, since you already have a reliable sexual outlet in yourself.

Using solo sex as a way to maintain your own erotic energy is a fantastic, safe, and pleasurable practice. We have bodies that desire pleasure, and in the absence of sexual partners we can give that pleasure to ourselves. It's quite empowering when you think about it. Cultivating a masturbation practice means that you recognize your sexual desire when it arises and tend to it. In other words, masturbation is a road map for getting from sexual frustration to sexual fulfillment all on your own.

We can also use masturbation as a way to explore how our bodies respond to sexual stimulation. One of the first things I discuss with my clients who struggle with getting what they want from partnered sex is masturbation. Most of us have ways that we enjoy receiving pleasure, no matter who is doing the touching. Knowing your own body and what it likes is crucial to having the best sex possible, because if you don't know how to please yourself, how can you show someone else how to please you? Knowing what turns you on and being super familiar with your own body makes communicating your needs much easier.

CREATING A SELF-PLEASURE RITUAL

Centering your own pleasure can be a fun and sexually rewarding experience—a gift you can give yourself whenever you need it. You may have some intense feelings about masturbation, so if that's the case, please take a moment to reflect on what feelings are coming up for you.

What associations do you have with masturbation? If you're new to it, how might you start to use it as a tool for exploring your body and desires? If you are already fairly comfortable with masturbation, how might you use it more consistently to support yourself throughout dating? Now, think about how you can extend your self-care to include self-pleasure. What would that look and feel like?

Simone and I worked together on releasing her feelings of guilt around self-pleasure. She believed that masturbation was something you did if you were desperate, and it made her feel weird to set aside time for it. She wanted to connect more with her sexual energy but found herself pushing her sexual thoughts away if she didn't have a partner with whom to explore them. I encouraged her not only to listen to those existing thoughts but to invite in even more!

As part of her weekly self-care, she found that she liked to relax in the bath. This was her time to unwind from the week and get herself ready for upcoming dates. I encouraged her to include self-pleasure in this routine by adding sensual elements to the bath. What could she add that would tap into pleasure by using some (or all) of her senses? She decided to listen to audio erotica while in the bath and then use a special oil blend for self-massage afterward. One thing led to another, and she reported that she let her own pleasure guide her through an amazing masturbation session. Putting masturbation into a self-care context made her feel freer to explore and give herself some much needed self-love. She found that she put less pressure on herself during dates because she was more centered and less worried about whether her date would result in sex. She also noticed that she was connecting more with people who were better matches for her sexually because she was more tapped into her own sensuality and could notice who brought that out in her.

If masturbation is something that doesn't immediately excite you, consider utilizing sex toys, erotica, and pornography to stoke your interest a bit. Many of my clients want to add these to their masturbation rotation but aren't sure where to start. Part of getting to know yourself and your tastes might be to start exploring sex toys. I love encouraging folks to visit a local sex shop, but you might not have one in your area. Luckily, there are also many websites that will deliver products right to your door in discreet packaging.

There are some amazing online retailers that cater to all bodies, orientations, and tastes. In fact, the femtech* movement has opened up more choice for a wider spectrum of bodies and different types of pleasure sensations. The development of more body-inclusive toys has led to products that simulate oral sex on a vulva and far more options for clitoral stimulation (without

---

* Laura Lovett, "Femtech's Sexual Health Revolution," *MobiHealth-News*, September 10, 2020, www.mobihealthnews.com/news/emea/femtechs-sexual-health-revolution.

penetration). Further, female-led companies have begun making erotic content that centers female pleasure, like feminist porn and audio erotica that lets the listener fill in their idea of what the characters might look like.

If you're someone who has shied away from pornography because of the lack of representation, unethical business practices, or just the sea of undesirable depictions of sex that one must wade through to get to something stimulating, you'll be happy to know that there are websites now that host content that aims to address these concerns. There are even user-generated porn and cam sites, where your money goes directly to the performers themselves.

With so much available now, if you want to try a toy or enjoy erotic entertainment, you can do so with the click of a button. These additions to your masturbation practice could be just what you need to make things more fun and exciting.

Take a moment to think about your weekly self-care routine and the things you might already be doing to take care of yourself. If you don't have a routine in place, think about when you might schedule some time for yourself. This can be time you use to relax, get centered, and connect with your needs. How can you add sensuality and sexuality to your self-care plan? When can you build in masturbation time? How might you tap into your senses to make it a fun and fulfilling experience?

EXERCISE: WHAT ARE YOUR BELIEFS?

It's time to reflect on your new sex and relationship beliefs. Take a moment to settle in and reflect on the following prompts.

What relationship messages and beliefs from your past do you want to release? Which ones will you keep around? For example, you might want to release the idea that sex can be good only in a committed relationship, but keep the idea that a long-term partnership is worth investing the time to find, and add that while you're looking you want to explore your sexuality to its fullest. Or you might want to let go of the guilt or shame that you've attached to masturbation, and keep your ideas that partnered sex should be fun and a source of mutual pleasure.

Is there a model for an ideal relationship that you'd like to aspire to? For example, you may have friends who exemplify the type of relationship you're looking for, or someone in your life who creates their own relationship rules that you really admire. Consider what makes these relationships stand out to you and what's appealing about them.

We all absorb so many messages about what we should want from dating, relationships, and sex, and not all of them are helpful. In fact, many of these messages conflict with our own desires for how we want to be in relationships with others and ourselves. When you take a step back from everything you've absorbed over time and compare it with what you actually want, you can start to uncover what is true for you. Using self-care and masturbation as tools to support yourself along the way can not only give you a boost as you date but also help you identify what you want sexually. Centering your own wants and needs is the best place to start. You get to decide what will make you the happiest, and when you center that, you are setting yourself up for a more enjoyable search.

2

Creating Your
Perfectly Imperfect Profile

If everything was perfect, you would never
learn and you would never grow.

—BEYONCÉ KNOWLES

work with lots of people who commit the cardinal sin of
dating: trying to be perfect. Perfect pictures, perfect job,
perfectly witty one-liners that say absolutely nothing about
the person they are. This has to stop, y'all, and I'm going to
tell you how.

But first I want to tell you why it's a terrible idea to seem
perfect in your dating profile. Your perfection does not lie in
how you look, what you do for a living, or how smart you are.
Your perfection lies in being a human who has a unique identity in this world—your own thoughts, hopes, and dreams
for yourself, your relationships, and your community. That is
what is most important to share.

Of course you want to attract people who think you look
amazing and are impressed by your CV or your many life

accomplishments! But are people who are primarily attracted to your achievements going to be able to see you for who you are and cocreate experiences (sexual and nonsexual) that make you happy? Maybe not.

Remember what you learned about yourself in Chapter 1? That is what future partners need to know. If that thought makes you cringe, that's okay. I don't recommend writing all of it in your dating profile verbatim. I do want you to think about how you can express who you are and what you want and believe a bit more. This will separate you from the hundreds of thousands of profiles that read more like perfect résumés and less like folks trying to find connection.

Another tidbit to remember is that your profile, like you, can and will change as you date. It doesn't have to be perfect the very first minute you set it up—in fact, it probably won't be. The trick is to start somewhere and revise as you learn more about the person you are and the people with whom you want to share your time. Think of your dating profile as a living document rather than something you put up for the world to see forever and ever. You can always go back and edit what's there. This can alleviate some of the anxiety that comes with creating a profile for the first time and, in general, gives you permission to change things up when you feel you need to.

By the end of this chapter, you will have more insight into how to make sure your profile is an invitation to your perfectly imperfect life, not an advertisement. You'll also learn how to convey what you value so that your profile attracts exactly what you're looking for.

GETTING STARTED

Many of my clients come to me in need of help with their dating profiles. They want better dates, connections with great matches, and more fun. I've helped folks use dating apps to attract the right kinds of sexual partners, find long-term relationships, and date outside of their primary relationships. No matter what the purpose, the practices we employ are the same: identify the right dating app(s) to use, tailor the profile to reflect what the client actually wants, and make sure that their values are clearly expressed.

Some of my clients begin their work with me using multiple dating apps. Others have never used online or app-based dating before and don't know what to look for when choosing a service. I recommend starting small, so if you have several active profiles, scale it back to one or two. And if you're just starting out, feel free to make an account with whichever app calls to you. You can always deactivate it if it turns out to not work for you. The key is to just get started somewhere.

I am often asked to weigh in on which apps are better, and I know that my answer of "it depends" tends to disappoint. But there are so many apps now that cater to different demographics and needs, so what works for someone else may not be the best fit for you. I've had clients who really thrive on the fast pace of apps like Tinder, Hinge, and Grindr, while others prefer apps that allow for more space to share things about themselves, like Match, OkCupid, and eharmony. Some of my clients use multiple apps, each for different needs—for instance, Tinder for general dating and Feeld for exploring threesomes. Social media can also be a way to meet and connect with like-minded folks. I've had clients who use Instagram for making connections with people they're interested in, or, once they match with someone in an app, they'll find each other on social and strike up a conversation there. The internet has given us the ability to make connections across the world, and apps like Raya don't strictly rely on geographical proximity for matching purposes, unlike other apps that use geolocation to match you with folks nearby. Raya might appeal to jet-setters, but not so much to those who only want to meet people in their current location. It's important to think about your needs and try to find an app that meets them, rather than relying on what you've heard works for others.

Take my client Cara, who was dating for the first time with an active focus on a kink she was starting to explore. Her other single friends were on popular apps, but she wasn't finding the kinds of connections she was looking for on any of these. She had started judging herself and questioning her worth as a dater because of this, so when we began working together the first thing we did was move her to a dating site for kinky people called FetLife, to better match Cara with folks who would meet her needs. Designed as more of a social-networking site, FetLife gave Cara access to a niche community that delivered not only matches that better understood what she was looking for, but opportunities for her to grow her network of like-minded people.

I've also worked with clients who were on "elite" dating apps like The League and Raya, and we decided to widen their pool because of the limitations of the communities that utilize those apps. Selecting apps is personal and depends on what and whom you are looking for. We live in an era when specialty dating apps are abundant, so if dating by orientation, religion, occupation, or cultural identity is important to you, do an online search for "dating app for" plus your interest and you will probably find something. There are also dating apps for shared hobbies, animal lovers, and, as I mentioned earlier, sexual lifestyles including specific kinks and fetishes. Trust me, if it's important to you, "there's an app for that."

Certain apps may have a reputation as being for either hookups or long-term relationships, but the fact is that hookups and long-term relationships are possible on pretty much any app you join. What's most important is that you choose an app that feels right for you to start, then test it out to see if it really matches you with folks you're interested in. If it doesn't seem like a good fit, move on. And remember, an app that gets your friends tons of dates isn't necessarily going to do the same for you.

My client Lili was dating across five apps when we first started working together. She was overwhelmed by the amount of time it took to sort through matches, message, and schedule dates, but she was also very underwhelmed by the people she was meeting. So when she asked me which apps were the best to use, I asked her two things: "Which apps seem like they have the most interesting people to you?" and "Which apps have produced the most promising dates?"

After answering those questions, we were able to narrow down her five-app habit to two: one that connected her with people who shared her Jewish faith and another that was broader but had connected her with a few great dates. With only two apps to manage, Lili had more energy for the dating process and was better able to vet potential matches. We then began to explore what she wanted and how to make that clear in each profile.

DESCRIBING WHAT YOU'RE LOOKING FOR

In Chapter 1, you weighed the pros and cons of hooking up and relationships. Now that you know how you feel, let's dig a little deeper so you can get some basic language to describe what you're looking for in your profile.

After answering a few questions below, you can refer to my suggested language to use in your profile. Feel free to riff on what you see to make it your own. Most apps will ask your relationship preferences and even use this as a way to match you with people, but I recommend stating what kind of relationship you're looking for (or if you're not sure) in the profile itself as well. This will give people a better idea of what to expect when interacting with you, and this transparency helps weed out poor matches.

EXERCISE: DEFINING WHAT YOU'RE LOOKING FOR

One of the most important pieces of your dating profile is often a piece that folks leave out. Stating what you're looking for is not only helpful for others to see if you're aligned on what you want, but it's also a time-saver for you. People who see what you're looking for and want something similar are more likely to try to match with you than people who see what you wrote and think, "That's not for me." If there's nothing in this section of your profile, then you have to do more work to find out whether you're a good match for each other. To help you narrow things down and get some language to use in your profile, think about the following questions.

- Are you looking for a relationship?
- If so, what kind? Monogamous or open/ nonmonogamous?
- Are hookups okay?
- Are you thinking about marriage, kids, cohabitation, etc.?
- If you're not looking for a relationship, what are you after? Sexual experiences? Dating around for fun? Seeking additional partners?

SUGGESTED PROFILE LANGUAGE

Now that you have an idea about what you are looking for right now, use the following as a guide for what to say in your profile. You can also use these phrases when someone asks you what you're looking for.

Relationships

- I'm hoping to find someone here to leave the apps with!
- Would love to find something long-term here.
- Open to making connections, but long-term commitment is the goal.
- I'd like to be in a relationship, hoping you're looking for the same.
- I'm a relationship person.

Hooking Up

- Keeping things casual.
- Hookups okay with me!
- Not interested in long-term relationships.
- I'm here for fun, but open to possibilities.
- I'm excited to connect with new people. Staying single for now.

Open/Polyamorous Relationships

- Currently in an open relationship. Looking to date, connect, and see what happens!
- Nonmonogamous and dating.
- In long-term polyamorous relationships, looking for like-minded people to connect with.

- Nonmonogamous-curious. Hoping to learn more and meet amazing people!
- Married and open.

Not Sure

- I'm open to meeting new people, dating, and whatever else happens!
- Here to explore and meet cool people.
- Not sure what I'm looking for, but I'll know when I find it.
- Let's start by meeting IRL and take it from there.
- Newly single and feeling things out.

Lili had been struggling with how she wanted to present herself in her profiles. She knew that she wanted a relationship that would lead to marriage and kids but felt awkward stating this up front. She asked, "Won't it look desperate? I mean, I'm twenty-four. I'm supposed to be keeping my options open, not telling guys that I have a five-year plan."

"But you *do* have a five-year plan!" I said. "Not everyone does. It's reasonable to assume that having a plan doesn't mean that everything will fall in place exactly how you see it, but it's important to give some indication of what you're working toward." She eventually decided that it made sense for her to be more up-front on the Jewish dating app but that she wanted to keep things vague on the other app. We decided to do an A/B test to see which approach produced better results.

In both apps she selected the preference for long-term relationships, but in the actual profile of the Jewish dating app she wrote, "My parents recently celebrated their twenty-fifth wedding anniversary. I'm hoping to find someone to do the same with someday." It was a beautiful sentiment that shared her relationship goals without coming across as someone who is counting the minutes until she gets engaged.

When we met a couple weeks after she had made these edits, she reported that she had been connecting with guys who seemed to share the desire to settle down, sooner rather than later. The messages she received after this change were more about what these guys wanted in their futures, too, and she noted that, qualitatively speaking, she was enjoying these chats more than what was coming through on the other app. I asked if she was ready to add this line to the other profile and she exclaimed, "Hell yeah!"

Though it can feel scary, putting what you're looking for out there helps the right people find you. Now let's do a deep dive into how you can inject this into each piece of your profile.

SELECTING PHOTOS

Dating-app photos are a great way to show who you are and what your day-to-day perfectly imperfect life is really like. Yes, you want to impress prospective matches, but you also do not want to give the wrong impression (e.g., a picture of you holding a fish when you literally only went fishing that one time with your grandpa). The scary truth is that profile photos are sometimes the only things people pay attention to, or at least they are what makes a person pause and take a moment to read what's in your profile. It's because of this that I like to think of profile photos as an invitation for people to see into your life a bit. The trick is to catch the eye of folks who are actually into you and the stuff you are about! So you have to show yourself being you.

Adding photos to a dating profile can make people feel exposed and vulnerable, so below are a few pointers to help you make the most of your dating app photos.

1. Use the Goldilocks principle—one photo is not enough, but ten is probably overkill. One photo of you in formal attire at your friend's wedding is cute, but having zero photos of yourself as you look most days is confusing. Aim for about five diverse pictures of yourself.

2. Center yourself, not other people. Use only one or two pictures containing other people so that it's clear who you are and who you aren't. You can also have all photos of just you!

3. Choose relatively current photos, within the last year. This may seem obvious, but people want to know who to look for when they meet you in person.

4. Include a full-body shot. Ableism, ageism, and anti-fat bias run rampant in online dating. Showing how you look head to toe can help limit your matches to people who see and are attracted to

exactly who you are. If you have a visible disability or physical characteristic that is uniquely you and you feel comfortable sharing this in your profile, show it in a way that feels good for you.

5. Show yourself enjoying what you love doing! If you're not an avid outdoors person, you can skip the photo of you on that mountainside. If you code for a living, show your work-from-home setup. And if you need to be in nature at least once a day, show yourself in one of your favorite spots.

I worked with Lili to select the best photos to use for her profile. She later shared that this was one of the most challenging parts of our work together. She was someone who hated having her picture taken, and she also stated that she was incredibly private when it came to sharing things about herself online. She had some photos that friends and family had sent her from parties and events, but they all made her uncomfortable. There was one full-body shot of herself from a friend's birthday party that she eventually approved. The rest of her photos came from a homework assignment I gave her, which involved taking selfies and asking her work wife and friends to snap shots of her while she was living her life. What resulted were photos of her sitting at her desk on the phone with a client, a sweet shot of her delighting in popcorn at the movie theater, and another of her laughing while playing with her friend's dog. She even threw in one selfie she took after getting a promotion. All of these gave a glimpse into her full life as a person with friends, a job she enjoyed, and pastimes that could spark conversation and connection. And that's exactly what they did!

Even the most seasoned selfie takers get caught up in which photos to include in their profiles. Remember, keep it true to who you are. You are inviting folks into your world. You might feel like the truest expression of who you are includes filters and if so, cool! If not, limit your use of filters and make sure to share at least one completely unfiltered photo of yourself. By showing the real you, you actually stand a much better chance of making great connections.

This was definitely the case with my client Sam, who had a ton of filtered selfies and photos of herself posing with friends and colleagues, usually at formal events. It was difficult to pick her out from the crowd, but on top of that she was overemphasizing her gala looks and had neglected to show how she looks 99 percent of the time.

"I just don't like how my skin looks up close. That's why I have so many group shots and use selfie filters if it's just me," she said. Sam is not alone. At some time or another in our lives, we are all subjected to unrealistic beauty standards that leave us thinking we should be something we aren't already. And most of us feel at a deficit when it comes to showing how we truly look to strangers who are primarily judging us based on our photos.

"Is there one photo of yourself that you like that isn't filtered?" I asked.

"I can look." She took out her phone and started to scroll through her photos. She showed me a picture her mom had sent from their vacation together the previous summer. "I like this one! I had just had a massage and was super relaxed and happy to be getting some sun."

"Great! Add it to the mix so that your matches can see that you look great with or without a filter."

*

A Note on the Thirst Trap

Thirst traps are sexually suggestive photos that folks share on dating apps, social media, and via text. They can be a great signifier of what someone is looking for (whether or not there is any text in their profile). Thirst traps can also be fun to use in your dating profile if you're looking to hook up or meet others who want to connect over a mutual sexual attraction first.

When setting a thirst trap, think about your best assets and how to accentuate them in all their glory. That means making sure you have good lighting, that your environment is relatively clean, and that you are showing yourself exactly as you would want someone to see you. Poorly lit bathroom selfies where you can see a lot of clutter or a toilet in the background aren't the most enticing. Remember that your photos are an invitation to join you, so how do you want that invitation to be received? This is a time to pull out all the stops and show off what you've got. Some folks prefer thirst traps of just their bodies so their faces can't be identified. I've had clients use one dating app for these types of photos and another app for their more relationship-leaning profile. It's up to you!

If you match with someone who has set a headless thirst trap, you'll want to vet them a little before meeting up to make sure they are who they say they are. Often they will be willing to share other photos on another, more private platform or via text message. If you set a headless thirst trap, you can do the same. Apps like WhatsApp and Signal provide end-to-end encryption to protect your message exchanges better than dating-app messaging will.

My client Reese was hesitant to set a thirst trap because, as an architect, she had seen not only colleagues on the app she used but also clients. This was not ideal. We discussed the pros and cons of putting herself out there in this way. Was the headless selfie the way to go, or should she move to another app? Perhaps she could start up another profile under a different name that wasn't as identifiable? She decided on a combination of a headless thirst-trap selfie or two under a different profile name. She was able to use that account when she wanted to hook up. This gave her a sense of security and made her feel less nervous, which allowed her to bring more confidence and flirtatious energy to her conversations with matches.

*

Remember my client Lili, whose goal was to settle down, even though she felt she would be judged for doing so in her twenties? She definitely wanted to focus on making connections that could lead her to a long-term relationship, but, like most of my clients, sexual chemistry was super important to her. She had had good sex and bad sex and knew enough about herself to know that committing to a lifetime of the latter was of no interest. That's when our conversation turned to her sexual values.

HOW TO PUT YOUR VALUES FRONT AND CENTER

We tend to think about values as they pertain to work and family, but knowing your sexual values can be incredibly helpful in guiding you toward the right kinds of people. When you know your sexual values and are able to communicate them clearly, you get to use a more focused lens to evaluate potential partners and experiences.

App-based dating can provide a skewed view of how many options we really have. The "good on paper" folks aren't necessarily people with whom we will have sexual chemistry. And the people who happen to find us physically attractive may not align with our values. While online attention and flirtation is flattering, for most people it's not the goal. Most of my clients want to meet someone and turn that into some kind of in-person connection. I help them use their values to attract matches who are seeking similar experiences. Because you know what's not hot? Realizing that you and your date are different in fundamental ways halfway through the appetizer course. It's a similar letdown when you realize during sex that you're both into *very* different things. These experiences are incredibly frustrating and can contribute to dating burnout, which I'll address later.

Defining your sexual values can help you narrow your pool of potential partners by broadcasting what you're really about. This can help weed out people who don't align with what you're looking for so that the dates you go on are more promising and even energizing.

EXERCISE: DEFINING YOUR VALUES

The process of narrowing down your sexual values may seem scary at first. You may have feelings that make you want to throw this book down and run, but bear with me.

The first thing I want you to know is that you are the only you out there. You have unique feelings and desires, all of which are valid, and you deserve the kind of partner(s) and experiences you're looking for.

Now, take a deep breath in. Exhale.

I want you to take a few moments to think about when sex was really good for you—I mean really, really good. If you don't have an immediate experience that jumps to mind, allow yourself to fantasize. Now focus on what makes this an ideal sexual experience for you. With whom are you having sex? How do you feel? What is being done to whom? Where are you? What time of year is it? If it's a specific memory, what was happening in your life then? Create a really detailed picture.

Next, browse the below list of potential sexual values. Are there words that correspond to thoughts you had about your amazing sexual experience? It's possible that many of these words reflect or relate to the memory or fantasy you just explored.

Acceptance	Growth	Privacy
Adventure	Happiness	Reciprocity
Affection	Health	Recognition
Authenticity	Honesty	Religion
Autonomy	Humility	Reputation
Balance	Humor	Respect
Beauty	Influence	Responsibility
Boldness	Justice	Risk
Boundaries	Kindness	Routine
Challenge	Kink	Security
Closeness	Knowledge	Seduction
Communication	Leadership	Self-Awareness
Community	Learning	Self-Respect
Compassion	Love	Sensuality
Consistency	Loyalty	Separation
Creativity	Meaningful Work	Service
Curiosity	Monogamy	Spirituality
Determination	Nature	Spontaneity
Equality	Openness	Stability
Expectation	Optimism	Success
Exploration	Peace	Surprise
Fairness	Physical Attraction	Travel
Faith	Playfulness	Trustworthiness
Friendship	Pleasure	Unpredictability
Fun	Poise	Wisdom

List adapted from James Clear, "Core Values List," https://jamesclear .com/core-values.

Now, pick only seven values from the list. These need to be your very top priorities. Things that, when they are present for you, make sex truly amazing.

Congratulations! You now have sexual values!

These words may surprise you, or they may feel totally in line with other values you have in life. Sexual values, while linked to sexual encounters, are usually not limited to the act of sex itself. In fact, some people view sexual values as relationship values—things that, when present for them in a relationship, make sex better and more exciting. This might resonate with you, or if you aren't relationship focused at the moment, you may see these values as specifically pertaining to the kinds of sexual experiences you want. Either interpretation is correct, and I welcome you to revisit this exercise every few years to see what values may have changed for you.

Review the seven words you chose. Is there a theme? Anything missing?

Some of my clients have noticed themes of "danger," "power," and "intensity," while others have stated that they felt things like "ease," "expression," and "limitlessness" were missing for them. Considering your list of sexual values, is there a key element that you feel sums up what makes sex really great for you? This is all information you can use later.

When my clients land on their sexual values, they are more able to explicitly describe what it is they are looking for with current partners and can better articulate what may have been lacking in previous sexual encounters.

YOUR VALUES IN ACTION

Now that you've determined your sexual values, take a moment to think about how you've applied them to your relationships in the past. Have you always acted in alignment with these values? Have there been relationships where you felt your values were not acknowledged? If so, how can this new knowledge of your sexual values guide you in the future?

HOW TO ASK FOR WHAT
YOU WANT WITH CONFIDENCE

You have done a lot of work so far to narrow down what you're looking for, determine how you want to present what you look like, and define your sexual values. Now it's time to put everything together so you can craft your profile with confidence.

After Lili figured out her sexual values were acceptance, affection, humor, monogamy, playfulness, reciprocity, and stability, she wanted to know how many of them she should include in her profile. I told her that bringing her values forward in her description of herself would be the best way to highlight them and that she could include as many as felt right without having to force it.

Below is what she came up with:

Lili, 24
Location: Denver, CO
Looking for: Long-term relationship
About me: Work hard, play hard, but also more play, please! You will always have someone to see the newest blockbuster movie with, even the awful ones. I'm super affectionate but with a dry sense of humor that can really throw people off. Ask me about my newest cooking gadget purchase or tell me about yours. My parents recently celebrated their twenty-fifth wedding anniversary. I'm hoping to find someone to do the same with someday, but also open to something fun for the moment.

The above may not read like it's asking much, but it is, and that's the goal! Lili is asking for folks who will appreciate her humorous and affectionate ways. She's asking for someone who is commitment-minded to reach out to her and spark up a conversation, but she also shares her playful side that is up for a fun fling. She is asking each person who reads her profile to see that she knows herself and what she wants and that she isn't afraid to share that in the interest of finding her best matches.

Here are a couple other profile examples that incorporate sexual values and make what the person is looking for crystal clear.

Khabira, 43
Location: Citizen of the world
Looking for: Play partners
About me: Open, kinky, and looking for folks who are active in the BDSM community here. I recently moved to the area and will be here for the next year for work. I'm hoping to meet other self-aware kinksters who are respectful, creative, and kind.

Khabira's profile shows that she is interested in not only meeting new people but also becoming part of a larger kink community while she's living in this new city. She expects a certain level of respect and self-awareness from partners. This will definitely resonate with folks in that community who want to make similar connections.

Jack, 37
Location: Madison, WI
Looking for: Not sure, but I'll know it when I see it
About me: I'm a teacher by day and an avid reader the rest of my waking hours. I'm open to meeting folks who can give and receive in equal measure. I'm shy at first, but don't be fooled! I can banter for hours with someone with a similar curious mind. Message me your longest Wordle streak!

Jack is not shy about putting his bookish ways forward in the interest of meeting folks and seeing where things go. The people he matches with will likely identify, and if not, they might be interested to learn more about him because of his emphasis on equal partnership and reciprocity.

In each of the above examples, the person has taken time to concisely describe what's ultimately driving them to date. They also give key information about themself and what they're about. We'll talk later on about how specifics can really help the right people find you, and how you don't have to write much to convey your unique desires.

Take a moment to put together a few sentences that incorporate what you're looking for and your values. Below are a few suggestions to get you started.

I really value _____

I'm looking for someone who _____
_____

The most important thing to know about me is _____
_____

*

Need-to-Know Basis

Some clients ask me how to navigate disclosing sensitive information while dating, like mental or general health concerns, a history of trauma, a disability, or a sexually transmitted infection. Many feel that certain parts of their life should be kept private and only shared on a need-to-know basis. Others want everything out there right at the beginning so their potential matches know exactly what they're working with. Neither approach is wrong. If you have a health concern that may impact your sex and dating experience, it's good to think about what aspects you are okay with including in your profile or even sharing with people you're casually seeing. Each of us has our own boundaries.

These areas of dating are tough to navigate, so it's good to think about when and how you would like to disclose certain personal information. When it comes to STI prevention, it's great public health practice to always use a barrier method when having sex that could put you or your partner at risk. But some STIs can be transmitted through skin-to-skin contact even if you're using a barrier method. One common STI like this is herpes. I've had several clients who were really stressed about when to disclose their positive herpes status, and we discussed ways that would feel good and supportive for them to do so. One of my clients, who was dating primarily to hook up, decided that disclosing her status before meeting someone in person felt best. She also shared how she takes care of herself and partners by not engaging in partnered sex during an outbreak. This allowed potential partners to have the information they needed before meeting to hook up and made my client feel more at ease that the people she did have sex with accepted her fully. You may decide that disclosing an STI feels best after you've been on a few dates with someone and when you know that you're ready to have sex with them. Regardless of exactly when you disclose, it's important to do so before you have sex so that the other person has the ability to provide informed consent.

Another common disclosure I see in my practice is anxiety, which can really get activated by the dating process. If you struggle with anxiety, letting potential dates know that it may take you a while to get comfortable might help set you up for more successful dates. Or you might like to see how you feel with someone and let this information come up naturally. When it comes to disclosing an invisible disability, it might feel best to share this information when you sense that the person you're with is trustworthy or when it feels natural to mention in conversation. For some folks, it might feel good to share this information in your profile's "about me" section. It's your choice.

If there is something that you have struggled with disclosing, think about when and how it would feel best for you to share it.

*

CREATING YOUR PERFECTLY
IMPERFECT FIRST DRAFT

Consider using the tools in this chapter to create or edit your dating profile on the app(s) of your choice. When you have a draft that feels good to you, share it with a trusted friend, asking for feedback about whether the profile really feels like you. You may choose to incorporate their feedback if you think it's valid, or keep it just the way it is!

You are coming to dating as your unique self, and there is no one else you need to be. In fact, being you in all of your imperfect glory is what will land you the most successful matches. Knowing what you want can help you identify the best dating apps for your needs, and showing who you are on those apps through your photos and your values will attract the folks you'll get along with the best. You may have been told that dating is just a numbers game, but really it's about the quality of the connections you can make. Folks want to see who you are and they want to know what you're about. Your profile will be perfectly you if you focus on these things.

3

Just Putting It Out There

If I've learned anything in the thirty-some-odd years
I've been with my wife it's that transparency is sexy.

—LEVAR BURTON

Many people struggle with honesty when it comes to
sex and dating. This results in poor matching based
on superficial characteristics, and I would argue that hiding
the truth is not the best way to begin any relationship. Perhaps the biggest paradox of modern dating is that we have
so much freedom when it comes to self-presentation that
we can be our authentic selves like never before—or we can
be someone else entirely. So how can you be more honestly
you in your profile? That's what we're going to cover next.

I've worked with a lot of folks whose major roadblock to
finding connections that work for them is that they believe
they should be someone other than who they are, or that who
they are isn't enough. This isn't their fault. Most of us have
internalized a lot of unhelpful ideas about what will make us
more desirable, lovable, fuckable, or "marriage material." It's

not surprising, then, that people choose to lie or obscure their true selves in dating.

What is so hard about online dating is that it's almost impossible to tell the people who are actually being honest from the people who aren't. But because you can't control what other people do, you can only try to be as open and honest as you can, knowing that it will deliver better matches for you. I know this is true because, time and time again, when my clients start embracing their truths, it results in higher quality matches and dates and more promising connections.

In this chapter, I want to help you embrace your true self. You hopefully have already started to do this by recognizing where you've come from, what you're looking for, and what you value. But putting it all out there for the world to see isn't always easy.

Take Alden, for instance. When we met, she was grappling with how to express her sexual desires in her dating profile without alienating people who were looking for long-term relationships. She wanted to build something lasting and didn't know if she could have the kind of sex she wanted with a long-term partner. The truth that she came to know about herself was that she preferred kinky sex, specifically as a submissive. At first, she didn't identify this way or use that language. "I'm just so bored by the people I meet online. It feels like a waste of time if I get all dressed up and excited, and then I meet my date in person and even if we have a lot in common to talk about I lose interest after we have sex."

Alden and I spent a lot of time discussing what she felt was missing from the sexual dynamic with her partners. Had she ever had the type of sex she wanted to have? What was it about these experiences that made sex good for her? She was able to pinpoint a few qualities that, without fail, were exciting enough for her to want more: power play that involved being told what to do, being restrained, and the use of language that put her in a submissive role.

When we looked at her current dating profile, there was absolutely nothing there to indicate that she was interested in this type of sexual dynamic (by the way, lots of people are). In fact, there wasn't much of Alden's truth in there at all! Because she was afraid of saying what she really needed, she didn't say much of anything about herself. Her profile consisted of a couple cute photos and an "about me" section that read "My best friend told me I should start an account so here I am." This was what was keeping her from meeting anyone who could deliver what she now knew she needed to be sexually fulfilled. There was nothing there for someone to latch on to and ask her about. There was also no sign of who she was or what she was looking for to help potential matches determine if they would be a good fit for her.

By now, I hope you have created or edited an existing profile that reflects who you really are. Take a moment to think about whether what you have in your profile is really you or if it is some scaled-back or exaggerated version of yourself that you think is more palatable. If it's the latter, I urge you to put at least one piece of information that is uniquely you in there right now. Trust me, it will make a difference.

SHARING THE TRUE YOU

How would it feel to be with someone who really knows you? Envision what this would look and feel like on dates and in your everyday life. Does this feel scary, comforting, anxiety inducing? Take note of what feelings get stirred up.

Alden wasn't comfortable at first sharing that she was looking specifically for a dominant sexual partner. "I've seen my boss on here!" she said. So I encouraged her to add a few lines about what she was looking for in a long-term relationship and then add "D/S" to the very end. For folks viewing her profile who already knew that D/S stands for "dominant/submissive," she was signaling her truth. Anyone who didn't know would likely read the other pieces of information in her profile and perhaps ask about what D/S meant. This would give her the opportunity to engage more with people open and willing to explore this with her. She felt this was a simple enough addition that wouldn't necessarily be clocked by someone she knew, and if they did, it wasn't that explicit. I also recommended that she start an account with a dating site that caters specifically to the kink community. This allowed her to see that there are others like her out there and to meet people who could teach her how to explore this part of herself safely. Over time, she became more confident about her kinky desires and was better able to describe exactly what she wanted from potential partners.

CHOOSE TRUTH, SKIP THE LIES

Sometimes we think that our truths are limiting. I see this in my practice all the time, and it's expressed in sentences starting with "No one wants to be with a . . ." Well, guess what? Whatever labels you have ascribed to yourself that you think make you less than or limited can actually work to your advantage. Knowing who you are and all of the stuff that comes along with being you is truly a gift to the people you're dating.

Everyone deserves to be seen for who they really are.

You may have had the experience of being let down by someone who portrayed themselves one way and then turned out to be completely different. This could have been revealed when you met them in person or over a longer period of time. Regardless, wouldn't you have wanted to know these fundamental truths about them beforehand? It would have spared both of you the time, energy, and disappointment.

*

Common Dating Lies
That Will Bite You in the Ass

1. Age: Super common and so misleading. You are the exact right age, so tell the world!

2. What you're looking for: Suggesting that you are looking for a relationship when you really aren't is amateur hour. If you're here for something casual,

just say so! The same is true if you really want partnership. Inquiring minds want to know.

3. Old photos: Just don't. One current selfie is better than ten professional photos from your teen modeling days.

4. What you're into: Saying you're into things you're not to attract a certain type of person will not get you far unless you plan on studying hard so you can keep up with your date's knowledge.

5. Your upbringing and family dynamics: It might feel better to fudge some of the harsh realities of your past or stay vague about where you come from in the interest of "polite" conversation, but most folks will want to know who you really are and what made you *you*. If you date them long enough, they will likely learn these things anyway, so try to be as honest as you can at the start.

6. Your job: One word—Google. Unless you are super stealth on the internet, your date will probably catch you in a lie about your job before the first date.

*

BE SPECIFIC: HOW TO GO DEEPER WHEN SHARING YOUR INTERESTS

Being specific is one way that you can share the truth of who you are and attract people who are into you. This doesn't just pertain to what you like in bed! Being specific about your interests will help other people find you and give them something they can connect to. If you don't make any other edits to your profile, just add some specificity to each line you've already written about yourself.

Why? Because everyone likes music. I repeat, everyone likes music. Stating that you like "music" or "live concerts" or "listening to your favorite jams" is not enough! If you hate music, that would definitely be an interesting truth to share. Other than that, be specific about what you like listening to and why. You don't have to make a comprehensive list, but it would be good to describe genres, artists, or music categories that you really enjoy. Case in point: two people who love musicals and own the cast recordings of every major Broadway production of the last fifty years should probably meet each other at the very least!

When you aren't specific, you are missing a major opportunity to match with people who are into what you're into, share your values, and are looking for similar experiences in life. Below is an example of a nonspecific profile, of which there are literally millions.

JB, 33
Location: Brooklyn, NY
About me: NYU grad. Currently working as an attorney. On the weekends I hang out with my friends and check out the newest restaurants in my hood. I'm kind of a foodie. Oh, and I love listening to music.

Big yawn! We have no idea what kind of person JB is. We can assume they're a college grad because they work as an attorney, but what kind? We'll never know. Now, this might be something to ask JB about as a first line when reaching out to them, but it's not really a fun thing to discuss—or sexy, for that matter.

Here's a more specific version of the same profile (with a similar character count!) that makes engaging with JB so much easier.

JB, 33
Location: Brooklyn, NY
About me: NYU grad. Environmental and energy attorney working hard to save the planet! Ask me about my favorite vegetarian restaurants. If you like jazz and all things Wu-Tang hit me up. Looking for LTR.

This is a much better depiction of JB. We know that they're an environmentalist who likes jazz and hip-hop. We even now know that they're here to make connections that lead to a long-term relationship. In just a few sentences, we have a better sense of what they value and how their specific interests reflect that.

Here's another example of a basic profile that could be more targeted.

Alaine, 22
Location: Montreal, Quebec
About me: World traveler who doesn't stay in one place too long. Seeking a companion (or two) for fun hangs when I'm in the city.

The above tells us very little about Alaine and what they might be looking for really. It's a good example of a profile that gets thrown together without much thought. You can be succinct while still giving people much more to go on, but these two sentences say nothing about what Alaine is like or what they're here for other than keeping things casual.

Below is a better, and far more informational, profile that is more likely to catch someone's eye.

Alaine, 22
Location: Montreal, Quebec
About me: I speak three languages but have no degrees. I travel as much as humanly possible (yes, even during a pandemic, though a lot less than I did before). I can't sit still for very long, but that doesn't mean I'll flake. In an open, long-distance relationship and looking to share my time with cool folks when I'm here.

Now we know a bit more about why Alaine, with all their globe-trotting, might be looking for local connections. Alaine has a partner they visit, but wants some companionship back home. This is much easier to engage with and ask questions about than the previous example.

Here's an example of a couple's profile you might find on a dating app or site designed specifically for connecting for threesomes or nonmonogamous relationships.

Sabrina, 35, and Jesse, 36
Location: Dallas, TX
About us: Monogamish couple seeking third for fun times.

The above needs a little more work if Sabrina and Jesse really want to have a fun threesome. They haven't given us much to go on, so people looking for a couple to hook up with might have a lot of questions about the specifics of this arrangement. Below is an example that shines a light on what this couple is looking for and sets them apart from other profiles out there.

> **Sabrina, 35, and Jesse, 36**
> **Location: Dallas, TX**
> **About us:** We've been married for ten years, have each dabbled outside of our primary sexual relationship, and now we want to start exploring together by having a threesome. We are very private and respectful but also quite playful and open. All genders welcome. We can meet first to get a sense of how well we vibe and go from there.

The details provided above give more shape to what this couple wants from their experience. They are new to threesomes, but not complete novices when it comes to non-monogamy. They also get to share their values and the fact that connection with the person is more important than a specific gender. This will be more helpful to them than the vague one-liner they had before.

Remember, being specific doesn't mean you have to write a novel explaining your personal intricacies, background, and things that make you tick. It means using the space you have in your profile to give people a chance to know a little bit about you before they even decide to message you. The details give you depth and set you apart from all of the other lackluster profiles out there.

USING YOUR TRUTHS AS
FILTERS FOR YOUR MATCHES

Some people believe in casting a wide net when setting up their dating profiles—keep it general and see who shows up. This is reflected in sayings like "dating is just a numbers game." We have all become accustomed to the feedback loop of receiving likes and comments, which can feel really good but doesn't necessarily meet everyone's relationship needs. Some people create dating profiles specifically for the purpose of getting external validation or creating digital relationships. They aren't necessarily interested in taking things offline. We'll talk more about these folks later.

My clients want to go on dates. Not just average dates, but interesting, fulfilling, soul-stirring, sexy dates. To do that, you have to narrow the search a bit. You've got to filter out people who aren't interested in the real you, making your pool of candidates small but mighty. And how do you do that? Put your truths out there.

That's what Grant did.

Grant had a couple apps he was using regularly to hook up and make friends. He didn't have a ton of experience with the meet-and-greet-style date, but he was ready to give it a try. We started working together after he had had a few troubling hookups that left him feeling objectified, and not in ways he was into.

"Listen, I know I'm in the minority as a gay Black man on these apps with a bunch of thirsty white men, but that doesn't mean I want to be treated like a conquest or as someone's 'first.' It's exhausting pretending it doesn't affect me, and I don't know if this will ever not be part of my dating experience." Sadly, Grant was experiencing what a lot of people of color are exposed to in dating—especially in app-based dating, where people feel more emboldened to objectify and fetishize people of different races.

I asked Grant when he felt the best when navigating some of the racist comments he received on the apps, and he quickly replied, "I told this one dude that I had zero time for or interest in being his first Black experience."

As he laughed, I said, "Great! Put it in the profile. It's true and it will hopefully decrease the number of guys messaging you who are looking for that. At the very least, it lets them know that you do not play."

We made a few other changes to his profile, including adding language about him wanting a boyfriend and photos of him on some of his traveling adventures, with his family, and at a speaking engagement he had for work. It read like this:

Grant, 27
Location: Chicago, IL
About me: Anyone else here a little tired of the soulless hookup? I'm not here to be your first Black experience or give you social cred with your brunch friends. I am truly looking for a partner to do fun AND boring things with! Second generation Nigerian excellence. Message me if you get it and wanna get it ;)

He started getting messages from guys who totally resonated with his truths. One guy shared that he had had similar experiences on the apps as an Indian American man and wanted to take Grant out to show him that chivalry was not dead.

When we discussed how these profile changes had resulted in more positive exchanges on the apps, I asked Grant for his take. "I was like, what the fuck?! I should have been less tolerant of the bullshit a long time ago. It just felt like what I was getting was all I could expect. It feels good to know that I can set my own terms and there are people out there who will respect that."

For a lot of folks, the swipe game of online dating is complicated by assumptions of what everyone is there for. I mentioned before that a common assumption is that online dating and hooking up are one and the same, so some folks believe that if you're on the apps, you're DTF.

There's also an assumption of white supremacy on the apps. Many people express a preference for a white partner or exoticize or other non-white people. Even when racism is more covert, it can result in folks of all backgrounds limiting their options based on what they believe is just a "preference." This might look like only swiping right on people who are the same race as you or who are another race that you believe is more desirable. On the surface, you may think these are preferences you've developed, but underneath, these actions may point to harmful stereotypes you have about different racial groups.

The world isn't equal in its treatment of everyone, and the experience of dating is no different. White privilege, colorism, xenophobia, and racism can all make dating apps feel like an unsafe space for people of color.

Take a moment to consider your past dating experiences.

Have you ever overlooked someone because of a perception of who they are based on their race? Have you ever given someone a chance because their race offered perceived advantages?

These are painful things to think about, but we have to recognize them in order to make changes. We can all make the dating world a safer and more fun place for everyone by checking in with and challenging our own assumptions. This is something you can do throughout the dating process by being more thoughtful with your swipes and recognizing when race may be influencing with whom you're connecting in person. Being more mindful with your swiping is particularly important because the algorithms on most dating apps will show you more of what you "like." That means you may be limiting your chances for your best matches without even knowing it. For instance, if you like people from a certain racial group often, you will receive similar choices. It's important to recognize the tendency to be drawn toward or away from certain folks and how that is impacting your dating choices on the apps.

Heteronormativity and patriarchy also loom large in online dating, making queerphobia and slut-shaming real issues that daters of all genders face. We each carry ideas of what gender means for us and often assume this must be the same for the people we date, but that isn't necessarily true. Gender, gender expression, and orientation are all very nuanced and sometimes require exploration for two people to really understand each other, whether they're dating or not.

Whatever your ethnicity, racial background, gender, or orientation, you may have felt frustrated by stereotypes and assumptions about what kind of person you are based solely on how people see you. For my client Zoe, dating apps were often a source of real stress and anxiety for this very reason. "I'm not your fiery Latina bombshell, okay?" she told me, exasperated by the details of one of her most recent dates. "And now everyone claims to understand intersectionality, but some of them don't have a clue and it's so disappointing!"

The truth about who you are can be interpreted in ways that are beyond your control. But putting yourself out there and even celebrating yourself in your profile can help weed out folks who do not want to take the time to get to know you as a full person. Zoe did a complete overhaul of her profile based on her frustration with how she was being misunderstood. She dates across the gender spectrum and decided that she would add more information about this into her profile, since she often got a lot of questions anyway. "I'm queer, divorced, and a mom. I don't limit who I connect with by their gender identification. If you understand that, great! Let's chat. Otherwise, educate yourself first."

It would be impossible to eliminate objectification, phobias, and isms from apps that base connections primarily on physical identifiers. Instead, the action I encourage is to lead with your truths and values. What is important to you? What are you here for? What should the people you date know about you? By putting these truths front and center, you can reduce some of the interference from folks who aren't there to make a real connection with you. The people who want to get to know you will make it through your truth filter. Some of them will be curious and might ask too many questions, but you get to decide how much to share and educate.

A BADGE IS NOT A COMMITMENT

Dating apps have started offering users the opportunity to add badges or icons that help clearly display the social causes they support. While this could be helpful for some people, I think it's a good idea to dig a little deeper when you see a badge that is of importance to you. It's relatively easy to add an icon to a profile, so you'll want to know if and how the other person shares your commitment to these causes.

Below are a few sample questions that may help you get a better sense of someone's truth as it pertains to social causes.

- I see you have a Black Lives Matter badge. How do you support social justice?
- I'm also super interested in environmental justice and food security. What drew you to those causes?
- Have you ever done any volunteer work? Where?
- I'm a big public health advocate. Where do you stand on vaccine mandates?

These might seem like totally unsexy questions, but with the right timing they can lead to conversations that will make both of you feel more connected and aligned. They can also help you identify if the other person is really tuned in to the causes that matter most to you.

EXERCISE: WHAT ARE YOUR TRUTHS?

What specific truths are most important when it comes to dating? For example, are there pieces of your identity that feel really important to share openly with potential dates? Are there boundaries that you have about how you want to interact?

What truth about your sexuality do you need to be more open about? Do you have specific desires that you can share or make a priority when you're searching through your matches? This might be anything from having your pleasure prioritized to having a specific kink or fetish.

How can you apply these truths to your dating life? Can you add them to your profile, discuss them when on dates, or use them as tools to narrow your dating pool?

You deserve to have dating experiences that feel good and affirming. Unfortunately, dating can feel so much like it hinges on the superficial that it's hard for your true self to be seen. Because app-based dating is so visual, racism, anti-fat bias, queerphobia, and ableism (just to name a few) can make dating incredibly unfun. Certain "preferences" might be preventing you from experiencing the best possible matches and partners. The good news is that everyone can challenge the assumptions they carry into dating and diversify their options by becoming more conscious of who they're swiping for and against. You can be a more intentional dater by sharing your truths and engaging deeply about things that are important to you. Your truths will create a filter that will leave you with folks who want to get to know the real you.

4

What Do You Even Want?

Desire is possibility seeking expression.

—RALPH WALDO EMERSON

Now that you have some ideas about what you're bringing to the dating table (that is, your whole, full, honest self) and you know what type of connection you're looking for, let's explore what you want to get from the people you date. This will be an important part of your dating strategy. Whether you're looking for something casual or your forever bae, in the end it all comes down to compatibility.

Sometimes it's hard to pin down what compatibility looks like, and the seemingly endless choices that online dating presents make deciding with whom to match even harder. Have you ever been enticed by someone's profile and thought, "I could see myself co-owning a cattle ranch," or "I guess I could handle being with someone who travels for work every other week," or "It could be cool to know what a documentarian really does with their time"? Online dating exposes you to a plethora of people, experiences, occupations, and lifestyles. This has been great for opening up the dating pool beyond just friends, people in your immediate community, and people you get fixed up with. However, getting too dreamy can derail your quest for compatibility and take you straight to Mismatch Town.

Going into dating with some idea of what you want from others can be really helpful. There are those of you who are thinking, "I know *exactly* what kind of person I want to date. I got this." I'll deal with you later! Right now, I want to address those folks who are thinking, "What if you legit do not know who to date? Like, at all." To you I say, not knowing what kinds of people you might be attracted to doesn't mean you can't date, nor does it make you less desirable. In fact, the people who know what kinds of people they like were once just like you! They had to learn who was out there, gather some dating experiences, and see how they felt. So, if you feel at a loss when someone asks you who's your type, please feel free to tell them the truth: "I don't know, but I'm trying to figure that out."

How much better would the world be if people were more honest about not knowing shit?!

I wish that I could tell you that in the world of dating there are two types of people: those who know what the hell they want and those who don't. But it's actually a bit more complicated than that. For instance, has someone ever asked you what you wanted in a partner and you just froze up with nothing to say, even though you had a pretty good idea of what you were looking for? You're not alone. Verbalizing or even sharing your desires online can be a scary, vulnerable act. That's why folks struggle with externalizing what they want or feel awkward saying that they don't know. It's a lot easier to either concoct some version of what we think we should want or keep our desires tucked safely away, waiting for someone to appear who seems to fit the bill. But as you know by now, making your wants known is a big part of attracting like-minded people.

The primary objective of dating is getting up close and personal with people who might be capable of giving you what you want. If that feels scary, don't worry! I'm not asking you to update your dating profile with details of how much sex you want, when, and how. I'm not even going to ask you to put your carefully laid out marriage timeline out there. What I *am* going to do is help you start to feel more comfortable asking for what you want and vetting potential matches using criteria that's based on what's most important to you.

In this chapter, we'll look closer at how you can identify potential compatibility, focusing less on the package and more on the qualities that you know will add value to your life. We'll also explore why it's okay to change your mind throughout your search and when to do so.

WHAT IS COMPATIBILITY?

Compatibility, put simply, is the degree to which you get along with other people. Is there a vibe or not? Some people measure it by how comfortable they feel with someone, others measure it by ease of banter, while others measure it by how good the sexual chemistry is. There are many levels at which you can assess compatibility, and I want you to feel comfortable using whichever scale feels the most important to you as you are getting to know people.

One assumption that folks have is that compatibility means that you will agree on everything. I think compatibility is more nuanced than that. First, it is highly unlikely that you will meet another human being who agrees with you completely on everything. And second, compatibility might be better understood by looking at how you handle the times when you disagree. Can you talk through these points of difference and get to a place where you might not necessarily agree, but you understand and accept each other's perspective? If so, that's a good indicator of compatibility, which includes an inherent quality of respect. And respect is a great starting point for any type of relationship.

There are going to be people you date with whom you're just not compatible for some reason or another. Earlier on, I asked you to dig deep and think about the messages you received about partnership and sex so you could decide if these assumptions are right for you in your life right now. I even helped you identify your sexual values. However you responded, you acknowledged the qualities that are core to how you perceive relationships, as well as what's important for your relationship satisfaction. Everyone you will date has these qualities and expectations too; you've just done your homework and have an awareness of them. But not everyone else has this level of awareness, or any interest in doing relationship homework. So how do you find people with whom you are compatible?

ASSESSING COMPATIBILITY

Tuning into how a person treats you and your time is one of the biggest ways to assess compatibility. It's easy to make excuses for how people treat us in the early stages of dating. It's an exciting time, full of possibility. Anything can happen! But sometimes our excitement clouds our compatibility judgement.

So often I hear from my clients, "They're just really busy. I think things will calm down soon though." And when I ask, "Are you prepared for if they don't calm down and this person isn't available for you?" the answer is usually no. This is a sign of a potential mismatch. Another common complaint I hear is about communication. "They text me all the time" and "They never text me back" are regularly invoked phrases in my coaching practice. These are also signs that there is a misalignment in how each party values or is willing to engage in communication.

Is it a bad match if someone isn't available when you want them to be or the communication feels a bit off? Maybe, maybe not. It's worth having a conversation about it, though, and verbalizing your needs. Sometimes these things can be adjusted and compromises can be made. But sometimes what you want and what the other person can give are just incompatible.

Quinn and I worked together for about six months, and during that time I helped them sort out their dating priorities. They have a very demanding job with very little downtime, so a big part of our work together was getting clear about who might be a compatible match for them. Quinn had been incredibly frustrated by every promising date turning into an emotionally draining time suck. Though they were clear that they were looking for long-term partnership in their profile, they weren't as clear about what that relationship would actually look like for them day-to-day. Once Quinn fell for someone, they would inevitably run into difficulty when they were asked to commit more time to the relationship. Their past partners always felt secondary to Quinn's job, and there was usually just no wiggle room for giving more than they already were.

Quinn and I had a lot of discussions about what could change, and since their work would often drain their time for months when a big project came up, stepping away to make more time for love was off the table. We then shifted our focus to finding partners who were equally busy or who just didn't have an expectation of spending more and more time together as the relationship deepened. At first, Quinn was afraid to ask for this, sharing that they didn't even believe there were people out there who would put up with their lifestyle. Maybe they could just keep coasting along and eventually someone would understand. I encouraged Quinn to put it all out there, as scary as that seemed.

The biggest win happened when Quinn added the following to their profile: "I fucking love my job, and I want a loving partnership too. I will make as much time for love as I can. Let's enjoy every second . . . I may only have a few to spare ;)"

The response to this up-front approach was overwhelming. They received messages from people echoing that they, too, were really busy, but that it didn't mean they didn't have love to give and a life to share. Quinn clearly stating their desire for a relationship that fit their life and what that might look like brought out people who were more compatible with their vision for loving partnership.

Another client of mine, Devon, was having a hard time deciding which communications she should take seriously: the person who messaged her "Good morning" and "Good night" every day but hadn't yet confirmed a date, the guy who kept sending her articles and GIFs, or the couple of guys with whom she was having consistent, albeit tame, chats.

We were working on her dating profile, but it was proving to be difficult to make the edits we had discussed because of her busy schedule as a nonprofit administrator and mom. One thing was clear: she really wanted to find partnership and was becoming very disillusioned with the wishy-washy communication coming her way. Sometimes it seemed like the guys were really interested in chatting, but when the topic of a date surfaced, they put her off. It was confusing, but she thought this was all just part of what dating was these days.

"None of these interactions seem like they energize you. In fact, it all sounds quite draining. What if you let them all go?" I asked.

"I'd love to focus on someone more interesting, but this is all I've got right now. I guess letting all of these conversations go would feel both freeing and scary," Devon replied.

"I hear you. I just know that you want more than a chat buddy. You're looking for someone to actually spend time with, and you don't have all that much time to go around right now. Let's start fresh. How about you update your profile with the new photos you shared with me and add in that you're a single mom by choice and ready to focus on building a relationship with someone? I give you full permission to let the conversations you're having with the guys you've already matched with die out in their own time, but it's time for some new energy!"

"I would definitely love some new energy! And a freakin' date."

In our next session, Devon shared that after updating her profile she had matched with a couple new people and scheduled phone dates with them. "It's what worked best for our schedules and it's a lot easier for me to prepare for than meeting in person right now. Things should be calming down once a couple new hires are onboarded at work. Then I can plan for more in-person dates."

"I love that!" I said. "How do these new guys compare with the guys you were chatting with before you updated your profile?"

"For one thing, they both seem really respectful. One even commented that he thought I was a good mom, which, I'm like, I am, but 'You don't even know me!'"

I told her that I thought her new profile did show more of who she was—including a sweet photo of her playing with her son—so maybe these matches were attracted to that and were more inclined to move the process forward with her. Maybe, just maybe, these changes had landed her more compatible matches.

"I think you may be right. We'll see!"

Putting your partnership wants out there isn't just good for you. It helps others save time as well. There are fundamental ways that we all interact with the world and each other. When you say what you want and how you want it, you are telling others who are looking for something similar or complementary, "Here I am!" It's like a flashing homing beacon in a sea of wishy-washy profiles that say nothing about what they really want or what they're capable of in a partnership.

WHOM DO YOU WANT TO INVITE TO YOUR PARTY?

Remember when I mentioned that your dating profile and pictures are an invitation? If your life were a party, how would you invite someone to join you? You can ponder this as you flesh out your dating profile even more. Paint a picture, using your photos and words, of what kind of life you have and how someone else would fit in.

Is your party full of biking adventures and outdoor activities? Is it a cozy, intimate gathering at home with an elaborately cooked four-course meal? Is it an erotic playground? Or is it full of family and friends mingling together at one massive fiesta? You choose! It's your life, and your party.

DITCH THE LIST

Whenever I talk about compatibility and emphasize that honesty is the best policy, I know there are people who start thinking, "Great! I'll just write down everything I really want and then I'll get exactly that." If you're one of those folks, hold up! It doesn't work quite like that. Determining what you want is a process of refinement over time as you accumulate experiences. We all have to start somewhere, so having a basic understanding of the kind of person you want to share your time with is great. Just be prepared to get it a little wrong before you get it right.

Sophie started working with me post–epic breakup. After taking a dating hiatus, she was ready to reenter the dating world, but not without some major skepticism. Her disillusionment with online dating stemmed from the fact that she had met her ex on the apps. How was this time going to be any different?

Nevertheless, she persisted.

In our first session, she shared how angry she was that things hadn't just worked out with her ex. He was a "good on paper" guy, someone who ticked all of her boxes. When I asked her what those boxes were, she opened her phone to show me a note she had started in college. The scroll was real! She had listed everything from age, height, and weight ranges to educational, income, and retirement goals, in addition to what kind of a father her future partner needed to become. In other words, she had created a list that included past, current, and future traits of a person she hadn't yet met. This was her guy, and no one else would do.

First of all, let me dispel the myth that you can predict with 100 percent accuracy anything about your own future, let alone another person's! Second, who would want that?! The world would be boring. We would know who we were going to become and who would love us best and . . . actually that sounds pretty great, but it's just not possible.

I asked Sophie if she had ever dated someone who didn't come close to what she had listed, and a huge grin appeared on her face. "Yes!" She blushed a bit, adding, "I hooked up with this guy in college and it was the best sex of my life." They apparently tried to date seriously, but she had labeled their entanglement just a "sex thing" and didn't see it having any future potential. He just didn't meet her criteria. "He's married now. I looked him up," she confessed.

We talked more about what made the sex so good and she explained, "It wasn't just the sex. I felt like I could really open up to him in ways that I couldn't with guys who I thought I had to try hard for or who felt like a stretch for me." She told me that dating guys who she thought were long-term relationship material put a lot of pressure on her to always be on. Because these guys had so many of the "on paper" qualities she was looking for, she often felt that she was on the defensive, trying to prove she was a good enough match for *them*. This was even the case with her ex; he was just very smitten by her early on and things progressed from there. The relationship had ended when they both realized fundamental differences in how they wanted to live after moving in together.

Sophie and I worked on finding her dates with men with whom she could actually relax, men who were attentive and active in the dating process by trying to get to know her and not just putting her in the hot seat. I also encouraged her to see beyond the list to the person who was in front of her on each date. How do they show up in the world and how did that make her feel? She began to see that the feeling of being herself that she'd had with the hot-sex guy in college was exactly what she was looking for.

At first, it was difficult for her to sift through profiles without her strict rules. Should she be swiping on anyone who looked cool, anyone she was attracted to? For a time, I encouraged her to do just that so she could see how it felt. She had some interesting conversations, and even a few promising dates, but when it came down to long-term compatibility it just wasn't there for one or both of them.

In one of our final sessions, Sophie said, "I'm having a lot less anxiety dating this time around." She had peppered her dating profiles with her values, some of her big life goals, and the fact that she was looking for long-term commitment. "I think the biggest shift for me has been away from feeling like I'm selling my best attributes to the highest bidder and more toward feeling like I'm sharing myself over time and letting these guys open up to me. It's refreshing!"

Sophie was able to find that sweet middle ground between two unhelpful dating mindsets that my clients often find themselves in. Relying too heavily on her list made her question real connections she made, while letting go completely of any expectations allowed anyone with shiny qualities to hijack her attention. Sophie had attained what I refer to as Dating Zen: a state of dating where things seem to flow and you meet good people and enjoy the process while keeping your wants and desires in mind.

Some of my clients don't even realize that they have a list, but when we start talking about what they want, they share lots of things that are "off-limits" that may actually be narrowing their options in not so great ways.

Take my client Danna. She had been really boxed into dating people within five years of her age who were artists of all sorts. She had a lot of mistrust for folks in certain types of professions, like banking or tech, even though some of her close friends were in these fields.

"What am I going to have in common with a tech bro?" she asked, exasperated, in one of our early sessions. "I just can't see how we would be compatible."

"So you've found that you get along best with artists?" I asked.

"Yes and no. The dream would be to find someone who is creative and can understand my work. People with regular nine-to-fives don't really get the whole 'visual artist' thing. At least that's been my experience. The problem is that a lot of the men I connect with through art aren't in a similar place when it comes to settling down. I was lucky and caught a break early in my career. Not that it's easy, but I'm not scraping by anymore. But people in the art world who are at my level are kind of insufferable to be around sometimes. So I haven't yet met that right person who can understand me, who wants the same things for their future, and who I don't hate talking to."

Danna was describing something really common. It's easy to get fixated on the specific characteristics of a person who you think will complement you, make your life easier, or help you create the ultimate power couple. So easy that it's taken as a given that your future partner will have a certain type of job, come from a certain background, and be a specific age or astrological sign. But these assumptions might actually be holding you back from meeting people with whom you'd get along exceptionally well.

Danna and I talked about whether she'd had the experience of dating someone who she felt really and truly understood her, something that through the course of our work together came up again and again as something she was looking for. She said she hadn't. Some of her exes were really inspiring for her and they had even collaborated on projects together, which enriched her life tremendously, but she hadn't experienced being with someone who she felt was really there for her emotionally and connected with her on a deeper level outside of art. In hindsight, it was all kind of surface.

One day, she shared her updated profile with me. She had opened up her dating age range to include folks five years younger and five years older. She also added a line that invited people who weren't artists to chat her up, in her own humorous way. It read: "I'm one of those rare souls who has made a solid career being an artist. I'm eccentric, but actually want really normie things like a house and kids and all that stuff. If this intrigues you, feel free to reach out. You don't have to be a working artist, but a working knowledge of the art world is a huge plus!"

This shift for Danna was enormous, and it opened her up to several intriguing matches. She even told me that she was meeting up with someone who had attended the same art school as her, but who had pivoted careers and ended up . . . in tech. "This should be interesting! I would have completely written this guy off because he only lists the school he went to for his master's and his position as a data scientist. He reached out to tell me that we had gone to the same school, and we found out that he graduated a few years before I started there. We already have had some great conversations, and this is the first date that I've been excited for in a while!"

So here's the deal: ditch the list. Your desires are way bigger and better than some bullet points you came up with five years ago, or some criteria that you think have to be met for you to be happy! In many ways, defining what is "right" for you in black and white or having rules about who you will and won't date robs you of possibilities and people who will exceed anything you could have imagined. The key is to stay open without letting go of what you're truly after.

This isn't about lowering your standards or accepting less than what you deserve. It's about being open to your *best* matches and allowing yourself to be fully present for whoever shows up for you. Think less interview, more rendezvous, and you may be surprised by the outcome.

EXERCISE: CREATING A DATING MANTRA

Staying present for the situations and people that dating presents you isn't easy. In fact, it's common to feel a bit adrift. Many of my clients benefit from having a dating mantra that they can refer back to in times of need. A mantra can be a word, phrase, or sound that evokes how you want to feel. It's something to hold on to when the dating process feels overwhelming or if you are starting to feel a bit lost.

The most successful mantras are those that express a core thought or idea you want to guide your energy.

Here are some examples of dating mantras to try:

- I'm here for love/sex/connection/the memes/banter.
- My person is out there/My people are out there.

- Let's enjoy ourselves!
- Stay open. Stay true.
- Partnership/great sex awaits me.

Using your mantra can help you to stay focused on the task at hand and bring you back to reality when you get off track. When should you invoke your mantra?

- When you open your dating app(s) and begin matching
- When messaging prospective matches
- When you get ready for dates
- In the middle of a date (though you may want to do this silently)

Not sure if a mantra is right for you? Some of my clients opt for listening to a song or a playlist to help get them in a good headspace when they feel overwhelmed. One of my clients created a playlist of hip-hop and pop songs that boosted her confidence as she listened on her way to dates. Another client opted for more bedroom bangers that allowed them to tap into their sexual energy. There are some great playlists on music-streaming platforms you can use, or you can create your own like my clients did. If you decide to create your own playlist, be sure to pick songs that evoke how you want to feel on your dates or that provide some sexual inspiration. There might be one artist you love, who always puts you in a good mood. Whatever you decide, listen to your playlist whenever you need a motivational boost or mindset shift.

HOW TO PRIORITIZE COMPETING DESIRES

A common experience my clients have is juggling competing desires while moving through the dating process. They want to hook up with someone but they are *supposed* to be looking for their next love. Sometimes it's the opposite: they're looking for sexual experiences but then someone makes them feel all kinds of *feelings*. Ugh!

You may have set a pretty strong intention when you started dating. Unfortunately, knowing what you're looking for doesn't guarantee that you'll get it on your timeline. But guess what? You don't have to feel guilty. That's right! I'm giving you full permission to explore the connections that come your way to their fullest. This flies in the face of the sex-negative messaging to limit the number of people you sleep with or not indulge in "frivolity" while in pursuit of something "higher," like love. It also allows you to follow wherever your dating life takes you. Anyone who has dated for a while will tell you that sometimes following your gut or letting things happen organically can be truly rewarding.

I want to affirm that it's okay to change your mind and do what you think is right for you in the moment—you literally only live once. Rolling with experiences that you're excited to pursue can be a lot of fun. It can also help you return to your original quest more invigorated and sure-footed. If nothing else, you will have gathered some good stories!

What tends to happen when you show up as your full self in dating is that you attract a lot of interesting folks who might be super fun to hang out with even though they aren't exactly what you're looking for. This isn't a bad thing. You just have to determine if these people are compatible with what you want *at that moment*.

Here are some common examples of people who may not be what you're looking for but could be interesting for the time being.

The Gift, aka "Sex Buddy"

These people may not be long-term-partner material for any number of reasons, but they help us explore our carnal desires. Many of my clients take what they learned from their Gift relationships and apply them to their expectations of future partners and LTRs.

The Welcome Distraction, aka "Gives Good Chat"

While you're waiting for someone you're more attracted to or who seems like a better fit with your sexual values, these folks supply the *best* memes, GIFs, and banter you could ask for! Count on them for a midday guffaw—you've earned it.

The Uh-Oh, aka "Emo Rollercoaster"

Just trying to keep things light? These people will show up to inspire you to feel all the feelings. It's okay; you can let them hold you.

STAYING FOCUSED ON
YOUR RELATIONSHIP GOALS

There is huge potential for getting distracted while online dating, in the form of dreamy profiles and long-shot matches. Recognizing this is the first step toward staying focused. When you're aware of what the distractions could be, you're better able to identify when you're falling for them. Then you can decide whether or not you want to be distracted and act accordingly. There is nothing that says you can't follow your whims a bit; what's important is that you are actively making that choice. If your relationship goal is to find long-term commitment, but you happen to find yourself casually dating a few people you like all at once, it's okay to explore those relationships and learn more about what you like and what might work best for you long term. And if your relationship goal is to find folks to explore your kinky side with, and you end up enjoying a night of vanilla sex with someone you're just really attracted to, it doesn't mean you're destined for kink-free sex forever. Don't beat yourself up over it. It's all part of the process!

One way to keep your goals and wants in focus is to write them out. I know I said to ditch the list, but there are some things that are actually pretty important to have in writing. Rather than thinking about a person with highly specific characteristics, try thinking of one to three relationship goals that you would like to work toward personally.

A relationship goal could be anything from going on ten dates in the next six months to learning more about what you want from sexual relationships to dating someone who isn't your normal "type." Remember, the best matches for you might not be what you picture in your mind's eye. In fact, a lot of what we envision for ourselves in terms of future partners is influenced by internal biases we have about what a "good" partner is. Those biases could include limiting beliefs about what kind of background a person has, or their age, race, body type, gender expression, or even orientation. Depending on what your goals are, there could be so many great matches for you that don't align with the limited ideas you have. Maybe you set a goal to challenge some of those beliefs about who is and isn't a good match, so you can stay open to amazing people you may have otherwise excluded from your search.

Think about what your relationship goals might be for the immediate future. The next three months? Six months? A year? Set goals that center you! What do you want to achieve in your dating life in these time frames?

You might even consider marking your calendar with these goals. It will help you stay on track and be accountable for going out there and getting what you want. Having something on the calendar is a great way for you to check in on your dating progress. If, three months from now, you haven't achieved your first goal, that's okay! You can always adjust the time frame. These goals are really to help you stay the course and remind yourself of what you wanted to achieve through this process.

HOW DO YOU WANT TO FEEL?

We've covered how having specific ideas about with whom you'll click can be limiting. What my clients have found more useful is thinking about how they'd like to feel with new people.

So, how do you want to feel in your next relationship or with your next sexual partner? What does your connection look like day-to-day? Really imagine yourself with this person. How do you feel in their presence? How do you spend your time together? What do you get from the interaction versus what you give?

App-based dating offers us a seemingly endless stream of possibilities, which can be hard to navigate. It can also be difficult to stay focused on what you want from dating when presented with so many choices. The trick to finding more joy in the process is letting yourself stay open to these possibilities while remembering that you have a unique set of goals. Some of the folks you'll meet along the way will help you refine these goals, and some of them might just be a welcome distraction from some of the lower moments you'll experience. Having a Dating Zen mindset will allow you to accept these distractions for what and who they are. You can appreciate what they bring into your life while also recognizing when you've veered too far off the path. We all get a little sidetracked, but sometimes these deviations give us exactly what we need to keep going.

PART 2
DO NO HARM

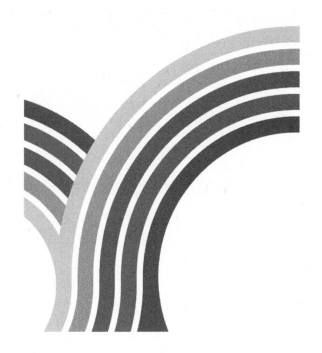

5

Just Who Are These Alleged "Matches"?

Love does not begin and end the way
we seem to think it does. Love is a battle,
love is a war; love is a growing up.

—JAMES BALDWIN

You've narrowed your pool of prospective candidates down to a small but mighty group of interesting people. You've matched with a few who seem to have particularly piqued your interest. Now you have to decide which connections you would like to pursue further.

Before we move on to how to vet these matches, I want you to know that not everyone you match with is going to be a good fit for you—not even after you've put in the hard work of speaking your truths. The algorithms that are working behind the scenes aren't going to know with whom you'll have great chemistry. That's up to you to decide, and sometimes you will get it wrong. This is all part of the process. It's called "dating," not "finding exactly what you want immediately."

Some folks have anxiety when it comes to communicating with potential dates. Sure, matching is fun and all, but the reality that some of these matches might end up in face-to-face meetings can feel daunting.

What are some of your fears when it comes to chatting with matches? Are you afraid you won't say the right thing? Is there a fear of rejection popping up?

In this chapter, you'll gain greater clarity about which matches to pursue and which ones to let slide. You'll also learn how to make a solid first move and start building connections throughout the messaging process. Part of having a fun dating life is doing the work of sifting through your matches to find the most promising ones. Being excited about the people you'll get to meet is one way to set yourself up for a better time IRL. So, have patience and read on for some pointers on how to vet your matches before you even commit to a date!

HOW TO VET YOUR MATCHES USING YOUR VALUES, TRUTHS, AND PRIORITIES

Sure you've got matches, but are they *good* matches?

What you want matters. And what your matches want matters too! When these wants align, that's when dates and hookups happen. The dance of dating is trying to figure out if there's something between you worth exploring.

Vetting is the process of evaluating each of your matches for how well you think you'll get along and whether you're interested in the same things from an in-person connection. You do this by sparking up a conversation and seeing if there's a vibe that energizes you. While you're doing your vetting, so is the other person. That means that one or both of you might think it's a good match. Sometimes you'll be energized while the other person is bored, distracted, or monogamously married. And sometimes you'll be turned off by the conversation you're having with someone who seems really into you. Know that you will likely be on either side multiple times, and that's okay. Because the reward for sticking with the process is meeting up with people you actually like who are really interested in you too!

Lark was at the beginning of this process and definitely had a steep learning curve when it came to vetting. She had always known that one long-term relationship wasn't for her and had identified as polyamorous starting in her twenties. From then on, she found herself dating about one to three people at any given time. She had developed a really strong bond with someone in her late twenties, and they decided to cohabitate. Other than the occasional fling, that was her primary and only relationship for about ten years.

When she and I began working together, she was in the process of figuring out how to date using apps for the first time. She had never needed a tool like this before, but between work and home commitments and a slowing social life, she didn't have many opportunities to meet new people in her day-to-day life.

"I don't know what I'm doing! I've matched with like fifty people, half of them seem okay, but how do I know who will be worth my time?" Lark had been messaging with every single one of her matches once she made them, for fear that she would miss out on someone really great. And because her primary relationship was open, she didn't have a cap on how many people she could see at one time. I felt from her the kind of overwhelm that a lot of my clients struggle with, regardless of whether they are casually dating, looking for monogamy, or in an open relationship. This sense of drowning in a sea of possibility can happen if you don't have vetting criteria in place to help keep you afloat.

The first thing Lark and I worked on together was adding some of her values (communication, humor, and stability) and truths (partnered and dating outside of the relationship for the first time in ten years) to her profile. We got really specific about the types of connections she was looking for, making sure folks knew that she was currently cohabiting with a long-term partner. I then asked her to sweep through her current matches and see if any of them listed in any way, shape, or form that they were interested in casual dating, in open relationships themselves, or okay with dating someone in an open relationship. This helped her narrow her matches down to about ten, which was a big relief.

We then came up with a few key questions that would help her assess her matches as they came in.

Here are some examples of simple yes-or-no questions for vetting your matches:

1. Are you attracted to them? Like, really attracted to them? Most people are guilty of the unenthusiastic swipe—it happens!

2. Does their profile seem to reflect values similar to yours?

3. Do you get a good impression of them based on what they've shared in their profile?

4. Have they listed information about themself that interests you?

5. Does it seem like they are looking for what you are? If it's not clear, ask.

6. Could you see yourself meeting up with them?

If the answer is yes to most or all of the above, go forth and communicate! Feel free to use these questions when you need them. You may want to add specific questions based on what you need to see in a match for it to be worth pursuing.

With fewer matches to manage, Lark had an easier time communicating with everyone. And on top of that, she was actually pretty into a few of the people she was chatting with. "I really like this one guy a lot. We chat here and there in the app, and he gives me these detailed updates about a project he's working on. We work in different but sort of related fields, so what he's building is pretty fascinating." I told her that I was really happy to hear that she'd found someone intriguing. "So, when's your first date?"

Lark paused for a moment and then said, "You know what? I have no idea if we'll ever meet in person." With that, she sat back in her chair and said, "This is what app dating is, huh?"

Yup.

I mentioned to Lark that some people may be perfectly comfortable keeping all communication virtual. And for a host of other reasons, not all of the connections she made will manifest into dates.

Here are a few common in-app messaging connections you might experience.

The Flirt and Fizzle

They're hot for you; you're hot for them. Things seem really flirtatious and easy right off the bat, then, poof! They disappear never to return again. They might even unmatch you!

The Sexting Buddy

Sometimes in-app flirting turns sexual, and you may find yourself in some salacious conversations. The other person may mention how good it would feel to do the things you're messaging about IRL, but they won't commit to a concrete plan to do so. Or if they do, they might flake last minute. Do not be surprised if they resurface months later for another virtual round though.

The Philosophizer

Big ideas, deep conversation, these folks love to stimulate your mind. That's about it though. They're not likely to meet up to discuss their thoughts on politics or history over an in-person dinner, but they will send you links to substantiate their claims.

Just Checking In

These folks are "busy," but they want to keep in touch. Who knows why?!

*

Having these kinds of connections can be fun if you recognize them for what they are. If not, they can be incredibly frustrating and feel like a waste of time. The key is to focus more attention on the connections that seem to be progressing, rather than on the ones that are spotty. This is part of your vetting process as well: Does the person seem interested in meeting in person? If so, great! If not, feel free to disengage if that's not really what you're looking for.

TIPS FOR BUILDING CONNECTIONS IN PRE-DATE COMMUNICATION

One of the top questions I get about dating is how to keep communication going so that you're getting to know each other through messaging, not just exchanging one-liners. It's not always easy chatting up a complete stranger and keeping things interesting. Add to that the fact that pre-date banter is one of the top motivators for folks to meet each other in person. It can feel like a pressure cooker sometimes!

My advice is to look for something in the other person's profile that interests you and comment on it. Whether it's a shared interest, culture, lifestyle, language, or hobby, having something to say about what they've written about themself proves that (a) you've read their profile (or at least part of it); (b) you have something in common or that interests you; and (c) that you want to know more about them. This tactic is great for starting conversations, but it's also good for when there's a lull.

You can also use their profile photos as conversation inspiration. If you notice that one of their pictures was taken in a park you frequently visit, let them know! Commenting on physical appearance is okay too, as long as it's unique and something you genuinely like about them. Everyone likes a carefully crafted compliment. Be careful, though, when making sexually suggestive comments. Coming out of the gate with a sexual comment before you know if they want to take the conversation to that level is not advised. Check the vibe first. If it seems flirty and fun, you may want to let them know what you think about their thirst trap.

Some people will give you lots to work with in their profiles (hello, truths!). Others will be sparse or have zero text, and you may have to stretch a bit to come up with something unique to say. Hopefully they will meet you halfway and not make you do all of the heavy lifting in the conversation. And if they don't contribute much, you may want to reconsider this match. Think about it: if the online chat isn't flowing or progressing over time, that doesn't bode well for in-person conversation.

In general, a good rule to follow in the first few messages is to keep it light and fun. If you're having a bad day, that's fine. You may want to wait to respond to messages when you're feeling more up for it. I remind my clients that in the early stages of dating—and that includes when you first start communicating with someone via dating apps—you have the luxury of choosing to engage when you're feeling your best. Once you're in a relationship or seeing someone regularly, they'll see how stress impacts you and how you are when you're having a low day. That's part of forming deeper connections. In the beginning, though, keep in mind that this is the part of the story that should be as fun as it can be, and you get to decide when you're feeling up for the task of delivering good banter.

Another piece of advice for those who are ready to date in person is to not let too much time pass without making an attempt to meet up. The apps are great tools for finding people with whom you might get along, but you'll only know if you like someone's full vibe by spending time with them out in the world. It's nice to have someone to chat with—and that alone can be a tremendous comfort—but if you want to see if you can make something happen together in person, then it's a good idea to transition the conversation to planning a date sooner rather than later. This sets an expectation of what you're looking for and keeps the conversation from getting too deep before you even meet.

SETTING GOOD BOUNDARIES WITH APP COMMUNICATION

Lark noticed a decrease in her number of matches once her profile was more specific, and the people with whom she was matching seemed more in-line with what she was looking for. She wasn't flustered by a ton of notifications pulling her attention away from what she was doing in the middle of the day. Instead, she was able to communicate with a few people at a time, on her own time. This was much better for her sanity, she told me, and kept her more present in other areas of her life.

We all have different expectations for how we want to use dating apps. Some folks like apps specifically for the swipe-and-match game, while others need time to get in a headspace where they can evaluate each person. Some people love the in-app banter and get a lot from chatting with lots of folks at one time, while others are easily overwhelmed and need to limit their engagement with other people.

Take a moment to think about what makes the most sense for you. Regardless of how active you want to be, think about how you can stay focused on the matches you're making. We'll discuss dating burnout and how to specifically manage your time later, but right now just focus on the boundaries you'd prefer to have with your matches.

Consider the following:

- How much communication do you want to happen on the apps before someone asks the other out?

- How personal do you want to get with someone you haven't yet met in person?

- Is it okay to exchange numbers and move the chat to text or another messaging app? If so, do you give out a primary number or use a third-party app that can keep your information more private?

- How often do you want to check in on messages you receive?

- Do you want in-app notifications turned on or off?

The answers to these questions will be unique to you and there are no wrong answers. Feel free to try something out for a while, and if you don't like that approach as much as you thought you would, change it up!

Now you have a game plan for how you want to keep good boundaries when communicating with your matches. But what if those matches seem to want more of your time than you're willing to give? Or what if someone seems elusive or unresponsive for long periods of time between chats? How someone manages their communication on the apps is a good indicator of how they manage communication in general. So if you're not getting what you need, make it known.

If you're not sure how to communicate your boundaries, below are some suggested sentences you can drop into your chats so that your matches know what to expect.

- When you can't talk right away: *Hey! I have a few minutes to chat now, but will be freer after 6 p.m. Chat then?*

- When you don't want to be on the apps all the time: *Hey, can we exchange numbers so we can text? I don't check my chats that often and I don't want to miss your messages.*

- When it seems like you've been chatting a while and you want to move things forward: *I'd love to meet up to test whether our banter holds up in person. When are you free?*

When you place a boundary on your time and how you like to communicate, you give the other person the opportunity to either respect that and follow through or not. Either way, you learn more about them and they learn more about you. There may be instances when your communication needs just don't align. It's okay to point these differences out and explain how the current communication pattern isn't working for you. Below are a few things you can say should this happen to you.

- *Hey, I'm not a huge fan of messaging and texting. I prefer more face-to-face time. Is that something we can plan for?*
- *I'm not comfortable giving out my number until we've met in person. Let's keep chats in-app for now.*
- *Communication consistency is really important to me.*
- *I put my phone on "do not disturb" while I'm at work and check messages at the end of my day. This is something that really helps keep me focused. Is it cool if we chat more before and after work hours?*

WHY MAKING THE FIRST MOVE IS AWESOME

Lark was feeling a lot more grounded in her communications with her matches, and she had come to terms with the fact that sometimes she would meet them in person and sometimes she wouldn't. She told me that what had been very telling for her was how people responded to her making the first move. She said she could tell almost immediately with whom she was more likely to meet up based on how they reacted to her.

"I'm learning that the men I tend to go out with either reach out immediately when we match or comment positively when I reach out to them first. It's so interesting! Some guys have acted really weird about me making the first move or even said they thought I was too forward when I asked them out first. And I'm like, 'Look, I'm poly . . . I'm not exactly a conventional-gender-roles type of person.'"

Making one's intentions known by asking someone out is a historically gendered act. The outdated expectation is that men ask women out, not the other way around. But what if you're not heterosexual or you don't identify as either gender and/or neither does your match? For a lot of folks, this very narrow view of what "proper" courtship is just doesn't work. If you're someone for whom these roles are important, then it's a good idea to vet for people who feel similarly.

In general, it's a good idea for the person who wants to make the first move to do so. But making the first move isn't always easy, regardless of your gender. Some of my clients struggle with initiating a chat after matching or asking someone out. I recommend that everyone try to initiate in a way that feels good for them. Think of it as an extension of sharing your truth. You want to know this person more, and to do so you have to express your interest in them and maybe even make a plan to spend time with them. When you boil it down, making the first move is simply letting the other person know that you're interested—that's all. What they do with that information is up to them.

Some people may not appreciate being on the receiving end of this type of direct approach. So here's the deal: those people will most likely not be a good match for you. You can feel free to release them back into the dating pool so they can swim on to someone who is a better match.

By recognizing that the men she was interested in either messaged her first or responded positively to her making the first move, Lark was starting to notice her red flags and green flags. These were helpful in her vetting process. Red and green flags are recurring events in dating that are signals for whether you'll be able to move forward with someone. How a person communicates with you, respects your boundaries (or not), and treats you in general throughout the matching and chatting process are all ways you can vet your matches even further.

EXERCISE: CREATING YOUR OWN LIST OF RED FLAGS AND GREEN FLAGS

While checklists containing must-haves for potential partners can be limiting in ways that might categorically exclude folks who are a good fit for you, red flags and green flags give you subjective criteria to gauge whether your matches are a good fit once you begin getting to know them. Take time to create two lists to help assess your interest in your matches. Red flags are behaviors or communication styles that don't work for you. Green flags are behaviors that help you feel comfortable throughout the matching and messaging process.

If you spot a red flag, it doesn't mean you have to cut things off. It's an opportunity for you to ask for clarity, set your own expectations, or communicate a boundary. It's good to know when someone presents you with these red or green flags, because this awareness allows you to know more about what you can expect from them.

Here are some common red flags and green flags that my clients have experienced while dating.

Red Flags

- Seems distracted or doesn't say much when we chat
- Seems put off when I try to initiate a date
- Moves the conversation to sex immediately when that isn't wanted
- Bails on plans last minute
- Mixes me up with other people they're talking to
- Can't remember key things about me
- Never initiates conversations or follows up when I ask questions

Green Flags

- Responds to messages within a reasonable amount of time given their schedule
- Asks me about myself and remembers what I say
- Commits to plans and lets me know when things come up and they need to reschedule
- Flirts well
- Listens to what I need
- Seems genuinely excited to chat with me
- Has a communication style that works with mine

When you have done the work of putting your needs out there, the next phase of dating is to see whether or not the people who seem attracted to these things are actually a good fit for you. There is a lot you can learn as you begin chatting with folks that will help you decide if moving the connection forward is a good idea. Some of your matches will align well with your communication style and feel in sync with your own rhythms. Other matches might feel forced, or you may find it difficult to get in a flow with them. Some of these matches will disappear for no clear reason. As you're chatting, keep in mind what feels good to you and what feels draining or generally like it just isn't working. Red and green flags can pop up and help guide you toward matches that feel energizing and help you address when things fall flat.

6

Dating Sucks. Or Does It?

Into each life some rain must fall.

—ELLA FITZGERALD

Contrary to what your auntie keeps telling you, dating isn't always fun! As much as I want you to get the most from dating and experience the maximum amount of joy throughout the process, sometimes it can feel like work and a tremendous time suck. We've covered a few ways to narrow down your pool of candidates and vet them, which can definitely help you spend less time on the apps and more time with great people. But this is just the beginning!

Dating is full of high highs and low lows. Anyone who tells you differently is either very lucky or has never used dating apps. There's a general trend of dating that you will likely experience if you stick with it long enough. It starts with a honeymoon period, when you're the new kid on the block and people are interested in you and reaching out at a steady clip, causing all kinds of commotion. This is typically followed by messaging with a few people and starting to go on dates. Fun! Or not so fun—it depends on how dialed in your profile is and whether you have chemistry with the folks you match with. The early stages of meeting up with people are usually a little rocky as you sort out your priorities and narrow down what and whom you're looking for.

Following the honeymoon phase, which can last anywhere from a few weeks to months, you may experience a lull. This is when you'll notice a decrease in interest, fewer matches, and fewer dates. At this point, you may want to swap out a photo or two to draw in some new interest. This is also a good time to evaluate whether the apps you're using are working for you. We'll discuss how to do this a little later on.

If you can ride out the lull—refining your profile based on what you've learned from the honeymoon period—you may see an uptick in interest and matches again. Sometimes how much matching you experience is related to the season. Most dating-app companies do a big marketing push at the beginning of each year to capitalize on folks who have res-olutions to start dating again or try it for the first time. You may have even been one of these folks! The beginning of the year is usually when the apps have the largest number of active daters, so this might feel like a boost. Summer is also a busy time for dates, as most people have more free time as well as the desire to go out and meet new people. You might experience lulls in early spring, fall, and early winter. These are trends to keep in mind, but they don't necessarily mean that you won't find what you're looking for during a lull.

The cycle of honeymoon to lull and back again can repeat itself over and over. It will be up to you to decide how much you can take and still feel good about dating. Because, while this is happening, you will connect with people you like who do not reciprocate and vice versa, people who disappear on you, and people with whom you share a mutual attraction—which for some is emotionally harder than rejection!

For seasoned daters, all of this probably sounds familiar and might be stirring up some anxiety. For those just starting the process, it might feel overwhelming, so pause for a moment to take three deep breaths. I'm here to expose today's trends in dating and arm you with some strategies to make it through virtually unscathed, more confident, and with some amazing experiences under your belt.

In this chapter, you'll learn how you can avoid dating burnout. You'll create your own dating schedule and learn when you should switch apps and when to take a break from dating for a bit. You got this!

WHAT IS DATING BURNOUT?

Dating burnout is a combination of fatigue and hopelessness that sets in after a person has been disappointed by their dating prospects so many times that they literally can't do it anymore. Most of my clients report some period of time in their dating history when they were on the verge of throwing their hands up and walking away from it or they were so exasperated by dating that they quit altogether—sometimes for years.

In fact, my client Kara reached out to me after recovering a bit from her most recent bout of dating burnout. She emailed me the following: "I'm not sure if you can help me. I'm forty-three and have been single most of my life. I've gone on probably two hundred dates in the last four years, and nothing much has resulted from that except a couple six-month relationships. My last attempt to date actually landed me with vaginal herpes, so now I'm really convinced that there's just no one out there for me. If you think you can help such a sorry case, I'd be interested in working together."

It's not uncommon for me to receive messages like Kara's, especially when the person has been trying so hard to find the right kinds of connections for them and continues to come up short. But I do not believe in lost causes.

I believe that there are many someones out there for each person and it is my job to help folks find one or more of them while enjoying the process as best they can along the way. Based on her email, I could feel how overwhelmingly dejected Kara was feeling about her dating prospects. Despite that, she was committed to keep trying with some help. She needed more structure to her dating life to keep her in the game so she could find what she was looking for sooner rather than later.

HOW TO MANAGE YOUR DATING SCHEDULE

One of the biggest factors that contributes to dating burnout is overcommitting—to matching, messaging, and going on dates. It can be easy to get sucked into the process of swipe-match-message-repeat. That's what the apps are for right? But spending hours a day, every day, on these things can drain your energy. Another factor is feeling like you're on an endless loop of first dates that go nowhere. Whether you're spinning your wheels on the apps themselves or on lackluster dates, dating can really take a toll on your emotional well-being. That's why it's a good idea to cap the amount of time you spend each week on dating in general and then break that down into activities.

Having a dating schedule does two helpful things. First, it gives you some parameters to work within that keep you from getting sucked into the Endless Swipe. Second, no matter how much time per week you set, a schedule serves as your commitment to the process of dating. Of course there will be days or weeks when you go over or under your committed time, but that's like anything else you put on your calendar. Knowing that you have a goal each week will keep you focused.

Below are a couple examples of how this might look.

Dating Schedule 1

Weekly Dating Goal: ~6 Hours

Monday: 10 minutes of swiping on lunch break

Tuesday: 15 minutes of messaging at home after work

Wednesday: 10 minutes of swiping on lunch break

Thursday: 15 minutes of messaging before class

Friday: 10 minutes of swiping on lunch break, 2 hours of in-person date

Saturday: 2 hours of in-person date

Sunday: 15 minutes of messaging

Dating Schedule 2

Weekly Dating Goal: ~4 Hours

Monday

Tuesday

Wednesday: 15 minutes of swiping and messaging

Thursday

Friday: 15 minutes of swiping and messaging,
3.5 hours of in-person date (option 1)

Saturday: 3.5 hours of in-person date (option 2)

Sunday

The first schedule is for someone who likes staying current and pops in on the apps frequently. They also don't mind stacking up a couple dates each week. This person makes a little time each day to engage in the process, but by only allotting themself a few minutes a day when they aren't going on dates, they aren't getting carried away. Some of my clients will set a timer for the amount of time they want to engage. This keeps them on track for the rest of the week.

The second schedule is for folks who either consistently experience a low volume of matches or who derive little pleasure from the whole swipe-and-match thing. They also can only energetically handle one date a week. Kara was definitely this type of dater. One of the reasons she had stopped dating before reaching out to me was that it was really hard for her to feel like she was making any progress. In fact, the more time she spent on the apps, the worse she felt her options became. But she felt guilty if she didn't at least check in every day. Part of our work together was helping her decide how she wanted to use the tools at her disposal and not allow *them* to use up her time and energy. I gave her permission to ignore the apps most days and just check in midweek for a bit to see what was happening. She was able to disengage from the process most days and then arrive more refreshed on the days she had scheduled herself to log in. Her whole mood about the dating process improved, and she felt more centered each day.

You might be thinking, "What happens if the people I've matched with disappear because I didn't get back to them in time?" Remember when we talked about communication boundaries? Your dating schedule provides a structure for your boundaries around in-app communication. You're free to check in on matches that excite you to keep things moving forward, make plans, flirt, sext, etc. What I want you to consider moving away from is overuse. Once you notice you've matched with folks, you can start chatting and then let them know when you are free to chat more if you don't have the energy right at that moment. Anyone who doesn't respect your time boundaries or isn't okay with reconnecting in a couple days is not likely to be a good match for you.

EXERCISE: CREATING YOUR OWN DATING SCHEDULE

Take a moment to consider how you might organize your dating schedule.

Given your weekly commitments, how many hours would you ideally like to spend dating?

Now think about your day-to-day schedule. How much time would you like to dedicate to matching, messaging, and going on dates each day? How will you allocate time for each of these activities so that you feel like you're making progress but not overwhelming yourself?

If you're not sure, think about what might *feel* really good. That might be five minutes of swiping, messaging, and matching twice a week or an hour every day! You can be as ambitious or conservative with your time as you want and your schedule allows. The trick is to try a schedule for a while and assess how it is working for you. Do you have enough energy each week to show up to dates excited, or do you find that you really have to motivate yourself because you're stretched too thin?

Once you've created your ideal dating schedule, how will you stick to it? You might tell a friend that you've created a dating schedule so you don't get too overwhelmed by the process. This will build accountability and keep you on track to meet your goal each week. Telling a friend about your plan can also help you when you're feeling overwhelmed. Your friend may notice you're headed for burnout before you do and encourage you to scale back on dating or even take a break. They might also be a great source of support for you throughout the dating process, whether you're in active search mode, needing to process your dates, or focusing on anything but dating for a while. That's what friends are for!

*

In addition to creating your own schedule, there are some built-in features of the apps that can help you avoid dating burnout.

Tips for Time Management That the Apps Don't Want You to Know About

1. Turn off notifications. They are there to suck you in whether you're ready or not. It's called "intermittent reinforcement" in behaviorism lingo, and it's meant to keep you involved with the apps at all hours of the day.

2. Use the paid features. App developers know which features make using the apps more manageable. That's why most of these features are behind a paywall. One popular time-saver that is worth paying for if you can is the ability to only see profiles of people who have already liked you.

3. Set it and forget it. With notifications off and clear communication in place with your current matches, you can take breaks from the process if you need to.

4. Move communication off the apps. As soon as you feel comfortable with someone, feel free to exchange numbers and ditch the in-app communication entirely.

*

WHEN TO CHANGE YOUR
PROFILE OR SWITCH APPS

You might find throughout your dating journey that the apps you're using aren't working well for you. Guess what? It is most likely the app, not you! If you've been very clear about what you're looking for, have some great photos of yourself, put your truths and values front and center, and you're still getting little return on your investment, you may want to move to a different app.

There are many reasons why an app might not be producing great matches. When this happens, think about whether you would benefit from moving to a more general dating app or one that is more specific to your needs.

Below are a few issues that could be interfering with your matching process.

Few to No Viable Matches

Tired of lackluster conversations or having trouble matching with anyone at all? Some of my clients feel disillusioned by dating because they've gone through all this trouble to put themselves out there but get few or no successful matches. I always encourage them to look into other apps that may deliver better results. Remember, there are many someones for everyone. You just have to find where they are—which might be on an app you haven't tried yet!

As my client Kara would attest, it's not always easy to find your people. She shared that she had run through six different apps over the course of her dating history before finally landing on two that she felt had more matches she was excited about. Her match rate wasn't super high, but at least the people with whom she was matching could hold her attention, and her interactions led to a few dates here and there.

Remember that dating goes in cycles, so you'll want to consider whether you think your lack of good matches is just a lull or if the app isn't a good fit for you. Try changing up your photos, particularly your main profile picture, and see if that draws in any new matches and invigorates your search.

No Interest in the People You See There

You may try apps—on the recommendation of a friend or through your own searches—that seem like they would match you with amazing people. But then you start looking around and no one catches your eye. Sure, there are attractive people, but when it comes to being able to relate to them, there's something missing. Some of my clients find themselves in this situation and assume that they are either too picky or their personality is not suited to online dating.

For these clients, I recommend finding apps that are more specific to their interests or sexual desires and switching over. This usually leads them to apps or dating sites where they feel less like an outsider in this vast dating world.

Catfishing

Something really odd was happening to Kara on one dating app she was using. It was designed to connect people with health-conscious lifestyles. As a former personal trainer and avid runner, she had gravitated toward this app when she was looking for a more health-conscious dating pool. It seemed natural to use an app that allowed her to build connections based on a common lifestyle. She met some interesting people there and had lots of chats about daily workout regimens and running goals, but she also matched with several people who turned out to be scammers. She noticed that these tended to be people who claimed that they were from another country and had recently relocated to her state, but that they split their time between the two locations. As a polyglot and world traveler herself, Kara appreciated connecting with these alleged globe-trotters.

The problem arose when she would try to make a plan to meet them in person. All of a sudden, they would tell her about an emergency they were dealing with abroad and how they could use some extra cash to cover expenses. This inevitably would tip her off, but it was disappointing each and every time it happened!

And she's not alone. Lots of folks experience this type of situation, known as catfishing, in online dating. Catfishing is when someone presents themself online as one thing and then turns out to be someone else entirely, sometimes convincing their matches to send money, sexual photos, or personal data. Some apps have more of a reputation for this type of behavior or have no measures in place to scan for or report fraudulent accounts.

Since this was happening with some regularity on this particular app, I urged Kara to drop it and focus her efforts on the more general app she was using. She made sure to add lots of truths there about her lifestyle and health goals to help filter out those who didn't share her interests, and this helped strengthen her interactions on that app even more.

If you notice that you're experiencing a high match rate with fraudulent accounts, be sure to use whatever channels are available to report these profiles, but also consider making a switch. Your time is valuable, and the emotional toll that interacting with catfishes plays can definitely increase your odds of dating burnout.

WHEN TO TAKE A BREAK FROM DATING

You now know how to structure your time to maintain your stamina when dating, and you know when to ditch your current app(s) and try your luck somewhere else. But life sometimes throws a lot at us at once, and there may be times when taking a step back from dating is the right decision. You do not need to feel guilty for taking a break. In fact, a break may be exactly what's needed for you to renew your energy for dating in the future.

You may also discover new things about yourself while you're on a break. Your priorities may shift as a result of having to deal with other aspects of your life and take care of yourself. There's value in giving yourself this time and space away from "seeking" mode.

And if you've been using the apps to hook up, sometimes you just need a break from sex. I know, I know . . . Who needs that?! But it's true. Our needs and priorities change as we date, so if you've been using the apps for months or years for hookups and finding new sexual partners, you might run out of steam eventually. Taking a break from partnered sex can give you time and space to explore yourself more. A lot of folks appreciate the opportunity to shift from having an external focus to a more internal one. You might notice this coinciding with the seasons. Spring and summertime can be very busy times of the year sex-wise, but then things may slow down as the weather cools off and people start coupling up, a time of year known as "cuffing season." If that's not your thing, it could be a great time for more you time!

Before you decide to take a break, check in with yourself by asking the following questions:

1. Is dating/sex still a priority for me? If not, what is?

2. If dating/sex is still a priority, is there a way for me to scale back for a bit? What could that look like?

3. How long of a dating/sex break do I need?

4. Can I commit to starting up again when I feel ready?

EXERCISE: SETTING UP A DATING SOS PLAN

We've just reviewed the many ways that the dating process can lead to burnout. It's important to recognize these potential obstacles and build a plan that can help you stay focused on your dating goals. It's not easy to sustain your dating momentum, especially after going on date after date but feeling like you're not making any progress toward what you want. These times can be disheartening and lonely. We all need ways to help boost our confidence and get back to a place where we feel up to putting ourselves through dating again.

Take a few minutes to flesh out a plan you can turn to when things feel overwhelming or when you're on the verge of dating burnout. This might include taking breaks, deleting apps, spending more time with friends and family, or re-centering yourself and what makes you feel good each day.

Reflect on how you can take care of yourself when things get stressful. Here are some suggestions:

- Create a dating schedule and stick to it
- Implement weekly self-care that keeps you grounded
- Journal about your dating frustrations
- Begin or revisit a meditation practice
- Schedule time for friend hangs
- Dance
- Masturbate
- Take walks outside to clear your head

Consider the following questions: What will give me a boost when I'm feeling low about dating? What do I need to remind myself of when things feel hard?

Part of reaching your dating goals is recognizing what you need when things are really difficult. It's not easy to maintain your dating momentum sometimes, especially when you've experienced a lot of disappointment in quick succession. Dating burnout is real, and it can sometimes knock folks out of dating for long periods of time. But there are steps you can take to make sure you're taking care of yourself and giving dating your best effort while maintaining your balance.

Setting up a dating schedule can help you stay focused without getting too overwhelmed. Your community can be a huge support to you as well, from pushing you to recognize when you're getting burned-out to helping you destress. Remember that taking breaks from dating and sex as a way to take care of yourself and regain your energy is perfectly fine. In fact, it may be just what you need to come back with more focus.

7

Authenticity and Vulnerability

More than Just Buzzwords

Staying vulnerable is a risk we have to take
if we want to experience connection.

—BRENÉ BROWN

We've all heard how being our authentic self and showing our vulnerable side can deepen our connections to others, but what does that even mean? The way we behave with others depends on so many factors, like how comfortable, safe, and seen we feel. And how easily we feel comfortable, safe, and seen with others depends on our upbringing, attachment style, personality, mental health, and possible history of trauma. If these are things you haven't considered about yourself before, it might be a good time to explore them through books and articles, or even by starting to work with a licensed mental-health practitioner. One of the biggest benefits of therapy is gaining meaningful insights into who your authentic self is, given how your history and life experiences have shaped you.

While being in therapy isn't a prerequisite for finding connection, it can help and support you as you encounter the awkward bumps along the way. A lot of my dating clients work with a mental-health practitioner in addition to working with me. Inevitably, dating stirs up feelings and thoughts about oneself more broadly, and therapists and counselors can help you put the pieces together to form a more comprehensive picture of who you are.

One last note on therapy: there is a pool of daters who prefer meeting others who are in therapy. The idea behind this preference is that they value having ongoing mental-health support and want partners who do as well. If this is your truth, feel free to add it to your profile too!

In Chapter 3, we covered how to present your truths in your profile. You got a chance to identify what makes you who you are and share your values and what you're looking for. This chapter takes things into in-person dates and explores how showing up as your authentic, vulnerable self and having empathy for others can ensure that you are seen in the best possible way and are connecting more deeply with your dates.

OUR VULNERABILITIES IMPACT HOW WE DATE

Take a moment to consider some vulnerable truths about yourself that you feel are integral to who you are. These truths go beyond your background and what you're looking for and are more about how you experience the world, how you relate to others, and what motivates you to date. Some of these truths may be listed in your profile already or may have come up organically in your communication with potential dates, like being introverted, being on the autism spectrum, or wanting to be polyamorous. Some of them, however, may be a bit harder to articulate to another person. For instance, you might find it difficult to address class or socioeconomic differences between you and your date, or to share how having a learning disability impacted your career choices. Certain things about us just feel particularly thorny to navigate, so either we don't bring them up or we let them dominate how we date.

Take Chloe's truth of wanting to have a child within the next two years. She had always seen herself becoming a mom, but she knew her preexisting condition would make motherhood more difficult, if not impossible, for her over time. This wasn't something she was comfortable putting front and center, but it definitely impacted how she dated. She focused her dating profile on the importance of long-term commitment and family. When she matched with people, she would make sure that they had selected a preference of "wants kids" or had written something that indicated their desire to start a family someday.

That meant that when it came to connecting, she had a pretty well-curated group of guys to choose from.

Where things became tricky was when Chloe met her matches on dates. She struggled with in-person dating because she felt that each new guy was a potential father to her kid, which quickly turned small talk into a discussion of life goals and questions about his timeline. While she was sometimes met with equal enthusiasm about child-rearing, she was so focused on that one vulnerability that she wasn't able to share her full self or see the entirety of the person she was on a date with.

She was becoming disillusioned with the dating process when we started working together. "If we want the same things, why doesn't it just work out? It's hard enough being single at thirty-five! For what I'm looking for, I don't really have the luxury of time that I thought I did when I was younger."

Chloe was brave enough to put herself out there and share that she wanted someone who aligned with her goals, but she told me that she felt she had lost herself in the process. Beyond this very important life goal, who was *she* and how did she see her relationship panning out with the future father of her kids?

There were other truths about Chloe that she had forgotten about: she was self-sufficient, incredibly charismatic, an amazing friend, and a community activist. With her focus on the time sensitivity of family building, she wasn't able to show up as who she fully was. She had detached from what makes her uniquely her, which often gave her dates a one-dimensional view of her personality.

One of the hardest parts of dating is showing up to each date ready to share yourself with another person, no matter how it goes. Things that feel close to our hearts can overpower our ability to open up, or we might even hide certain things that we don't want to be judged negatively for. It sometimes feels crazy to open up over and over in the interest of getting what you want. But it is this willingness to be vulnerable about all of the things that make us who we are that leads to just that.

*

Brave Acts of Vulnerability

Vulnerability can look lots of different ways and can manifest in acts big and small.

- One of my clients who wanted more sexual experience started to share with potential partners that she was a survivor of sexual assault. She developed a couple supportive connections with folks who were willing to discuss this with her and move at her pace when it came to sex.

- One of my clients had sex with someone she met online after a seven-year dry spell! When she felt comfortable enough with her partner, she shared that she "hadn't been naked with another person for a long time." This helped her partner understand why she seemed so nervous, and they were better able to find their rhythm together.

- One of my clients, who struggled with sharing how she felt with her new partner, decided to switch the blue heart emoji that she was using in her texts to him to red. He noticed and commented that things must be getting serious for her and that he was feeling the same way!

- All of my clients are choosing to make sex a priority in their life. That can feel incredibly vulnerable.

- Reading this book is a vulnerable act! Take a moment to reflect on all you've already done and the parts of yourself that you are letting come forward more.

*

What factors make it difficult to be your authentic self on dates? Think about when you've felt like you were playing either up or down certain aspects of who you are. What was going on in the conversation?

Now envision how you can respond differently in the future. How can you bring more of your authentic self forward?

QUESTIONS FOR DEEPENING CONNECTIONS WITH YOUR DATES

Meeting someone face-to-face for the first time, whether virtually or in person, is a universally anxiety-inducing experience. But it is one that is absolutely necessary, whether you're looking to hook up or settle down. First-meeting jitters are real and can range from slightly nerve-racking to painfully awkward. When you're in a state of nervousness, no matter how minor, it may be difficult to be your usual charming self. This is perfectly okay! The nerves will pass.

Remember the mantra you created for yourself in Chapter 4? Feel free to use this to ground yourself before any first meetings and stay present with your intention for dating.

The basic building blocks of connection are interest in and concern for the other person and a willingness to divulge information about yourself that will help them learn who you are. The easiest way to use these building blocks is by asking and responding to questions. This should be a fairly organic process, but if you find yourself at a loss for words due to nerves, feel free to fall back on the following questions to start building a connection with your date.

For Sex or Casual Dates

- What has been exciting you lately?
- What would you like from our experience together?
- Do you need anything? Is there anything I should keep in mind to make this experience good for you?

For Dates with Folks You May Want to Date Long Term

- What energizes you?
- When you have free time, what do you like to do?
- I noticed in your profile that you're into _____. Tell me more about that. How did you get into it?

Getting the conversation started isn't always easy, but having a strong beginning can make all the difference. Building connection is an active process. It's more than give-and-take or call-and-response. It's tuning into each moment and assessing how much deeper you can go. What makes you feel good, teaches you more, or draws the other person in?

This active, forward momentum is what allows people to cocreate experiences together. But what about when there's a lull or you're not sure where to steer things? Below are a few general questions that can help you, whether you are trying to build a sexual connection or go deeper into the conversation.

For Sex or Casual Dates

- Can I kiss you?
- I really want to move this to (my/your place, the bedroom, someplace more private, etc.). Is that okay with you?
- Will you show me where you want me to touch/kiss you?

For Dates with Folks You May Want to Date Long Term

- What made you decide to go on the apps?
- Ideally, what are you hoping to find through dating?
- How are you feeling so far?

*

Guidelines for Asking Your Date Questions and Responding to Theirs

- If you ask, be prepared to answer. Don't be surprised if the questions you ask your date are returned to you. If you ask someone something about themself, make sure you feel comfortable addressing it as well.

- It's important for the flow of conversation to keep things balanced. If you find yourself asking a lot of questions, pause and make sure you give the floor to your date for a bit.

- If your date asks you pointed questions, try to answer everything to the best of your ability. "I don't know" and "I've never thought about that before" are okay responses, just be aware that you'll need to take the conversation elsewhere afterward.

- If someone asks a question you would rather not answer, kindly tell them that you're not ready to address that yet or that you'd like to leave a little mystery for future conversations. Remember, boundaries are good and help you stay true to yourself!

*

DATING IS A PRACTICE IN VULNERABILITY

No matter what brought you to dating, the simple act of declaring that you are looking for someone else (or many someones) can feel really vulnerable. And it just gets more intense the closer you get to reaching your dating goals. A lot of my clients struggle with opening up throughout the dating process because, honestly, being vulnerable can be exhausting. I don't blame them!

We all have different thresholds for vulnerability. Some folks feel more comfortable experiencing desire, disappointment, anticipation, and rejection than other people. Some daters develop higher tolerances for certain emotions the more they experience them. They find that rejection stings the first few times, but then they come to understand that it's part of the process of trying to find the best people. This doesn't mean they won't feel rejection acutely again; it just means that they may move through their experience of it a little easier. Other folks will struggle with big feelings no matter how much they experience them.

My client Tatya wore her rejections like badges of honor. She felt strongly that, with each person it didn't work out with, she was getting closer to figuring out not only what she wanted but also who she wanted it with. Whereas my client Jax always struggled when faced with rejection. It took them a little while after each instance to muster the energy to get back into dating. While they processed, they spent time with friends who helped them reconnect with why they were putting themself out there, and after a few pep talks from their nearest and dearest they were ready to start their search again.

Let's check in for a moment. Which emotions make you feel the most vulnerable?

If you have trouble thinking of words on your own, review the below list of the eight basic emotions:*

- Fear
- Anger
- Sadness
- Joy
- Disgust
- Surprise
- Trust
- Anticipation

It's easy to see how dating could stir up any and all of the above emotions. Feel free to think of other emotions that make you feel vulnerable and consider when they might show up for you in dating. It's good to think about, because dating can be a practice of vulnerability and so can sex. Think about it: sex is probably the most vulnerable thing we do with others. We're literally naked and exposed for who we are. Knowing what emotional or even physical territory makes you feel vulnerable can help you communicate your needs more clearly throughout dating. Naming what emotion is showing up and recognizing you're in vulnerable territory can help you navigate these experiences more easily.

---

* Robert Plutchik, "A General Psychoevolutionary Theory of Emotion," in *Theories of Emotion*, eds. Robert Plutchik and Henry Kellerman (Cambridge, MA: Academic Press, 1980), 3–33, https://doi.org/10.1016/b978-0-12-558701-3.50007-7.

Aaliyah, like so many of my clients, was yearning for sexual connection. In the past, her dating experiences had been incredibly difficult. She was a survivor of sexual assault and had a hard time recognizing and communicating her triggers. When we began working together, she had been through intensive therapy and now met with a therapist every other week to check in. She had worked to understand her triggers and was ready to give sex another shot. She was interested in casual relationships but open if someone came into her life who seemed like a good match for long-term partnership.

The assault Aaliyah experienced in her early twenties made her feel incredibly uncomfortable on dates in the years that followed, usually resulting in drunken one-night stands or emotionally fraught sexual encounters with short-term partners. Now in her thirties, she knew more about what she needed from partners to make her feel comfortable taking things to a sexual place. She felt vulnerable communicating what she needed and trusting that the work she had done in therapy and with me would lead her to partners who would listen to and respect her needs. This was all new territory.

"How can I trust that they'll listen to me? Or, how do I know that after I tell them what I need they'll even want to sleep with me at all?" We worked on her dating profiles and she set up some vetting practices that made her feel better about the folks she was meeting in person, all of whom seemed attentive to her needs. Aaliyah had a lot of support to help her get through the more challenging aspects of dating, and over time she became more confident in her ability to select partners who were truly invested in connecting with her authentically. She had built up her communication skills to the point where she could sense when it was appropriate to share about her past experience in the interest of helping the other person learn about her and connect more deeply. Sometimes this happened on the first date; other times it happened after a few dates or right before having sex.

"I think I might be having the best sex of my life!" she shared in one session. When I asked her to tell me how sex felt better to her now, she said, "I'm just more me, I think— triggers and all! I'm learning when it feels safe to let myself go, and that that can be really freeing during sex. I wasn't able to do that before because I didn't know that it was okay to stop if I felt awkward or scared. I was always worried about ruining the moment."

For anyone who has experienced sexual assault or a trauma that makes sexual connection difficult, know that there are so many people out there like you who have been able to create great sex lives for themselves. It is usually a vulnerable process, and it will likely require time and some help along the way.

Even if you haven't experienced assault, sex can be very tricky and vulnerable. We could all stand to recognize this a bit more. And that's where empathy comes in.

HOW EMPATHY CREATES STRONGER CONNECTIONS

Knowing that dating and sex are vulnerable acts and that most daters experience some form of anxiety when meeting up can give you a bit of empathy for your dates. Empathy is the ability to understand and relate to how another person might be feeling. It takes the focus off of you and whatever might be swirling around in your head and gives you a chance to connect with the other person about their emotional needs. This is key to deepening connection.

Aaliyah noticed the people she felt most comfortable with (and therefore able to fully open up to and be vulnerable with) were the ones who showed empathy toward her. This, in turn, allowed her to build trust. She recalled this in small behaviors, like the time when she arrived late to a date because the rideshare she was in got into a slight fender bender. She arrived flustered and apologetic, and her date immediately offered her a glass of water, recognizing that she seemed overwhelmed. He sat calmly while she collected herself and explained what had happened, then said, "Oh wow, do you need anything else besides water? I know I get super nervous before dates, and then add a car accident on top of that? Thank you for still coming to meet me!"

Empathetic partners made being sexually intimate a lot easier for Aaliyah. She found that attentive partners would check in to make sure she was still enjoying herself, and if she ever got overwhelmed they would give her space and talk to her about what she needed in that moment. They were patient and had a vested interest in having a mutually enjoyable experience. She felt that the combination of noticing her emotional state, being clear about her needs, and having empathetic partners made for better sexual connection in general.

Something peculiar happens when you practice empathy for others. You may find that your own dating anxieties lessen over time as you internalize the fact that your dates—as calm and collected as they appear on the surface—are often just as nervous as you are and that regardless of how attractive someone is or how successful they seem to be, they, too, are fearful of rejection. This commonality makes us all equals when it comes to dating. Yes, some people will have an easier time dating than others. And yes, systemic inequalities make the playing field unfair for a lot of folks out there. But these are things you can empathize with as well!

There are no boundaries around who can empathize with whom. You don't have to have a direct experience to be able to empathize with someone and what they might have gone through. Empathy only requires you to imagine what it might be like for the other person and feel what they might feel.

For instance, men can empathize with women who have experienced harassment and understand that it sucks to be objectified, without having directly experienced this for themselves. White people can empathize, to some degree, with the mental toll that racism takes on people of color, without having experienced racism. Of course, you will never know exactly how someone else feels or how their experiences shaped them, so it's important to let folks share their unique perspective and stay open to what they have to say. If you find yourself having a hard time empathizing with or understanding what your dates share with you, you can always do your own research to learn more about the topics they bring up. In the meantime, active listening and withholding judgment go a long way.

*

Empathy: A Primer

The best way to empathize with someone and show that you want to know more about their experience is to let them share about themself first. When they do open up about a vulnerable aspect, you can say something like "That must have been hard for you" or "If you feel comfortable talking about it, I'd love to hear more about how that affected you." These statements allow the other person to feel seen and invited to share more without adding pressure.

Steer clear of making assumptions or relying on stereotypes. Empathy comes from a genuine attempt to understand the other person. It is not laying out how you *think* they feel before you get to know them or have information to pull from. An example of this would be saying things like "As someone with a disability, you must have felt like an outsider growing up," before the person has shared specifics about the nature of their disability and what their childhood was like. They may have had a very different experience than the one you created in your head for them.

The key is to listen, stay curious, and imagine how the other person might feel given what they've shared. This can make all the difference in your ability to build meaningful connections.

*

EXERCISE: WHAT DOES BEING AUTHENTIC AND VULNERABLE MEAN TO YOU?

We just covered how dating is often a vulnerable practice, and then added to that the fact that most people experience an additional layer of vulnerability during sex. There's so much to navigate, but when you are able to show who you are and have that met with acceptance and curiosity rather than judgment and rejection, it can make everything worthwhile. Take a few deep breaths and think for a moment about how being exactly who you are, vulnerabilities and all, is all you need to do. Just being you is enough.

How might you bring more of yourself into your dating experiences? This might look like ending things with folks you can't be yourself around, or sharing your vulnerabilities when you feel safe enough with someone to do so. It might be as simple as reading this book and applying what you learn to dating when you're ready.

Meeting people for the first time can stir up all kinds of emotions. Even if you feel confident in what you're looking for and what you'd like to get from the experience, showing up as your full self takes practice. To start, getting familiar with the hard-to-articulate parts of yourself can be useful. When you start to feel a connection forming, it can be moments of sharing these aspects that invite a deeper understanding of you. This type of understanding goes both ways. Your date may share vulnerable truths about themself that you may have no experience with. That's where empathy comes in. Connections grow stronger when both parties are open to hearing each other and imagining what the other person might be experiencing. From there, you can ask questions, learn, and open up even more.

8

You Can Have It All
(Just Not All at Once)

That whole "so you can have it all."
Nope, not at the same time. That's a lie.

—MICHELLE OBAMA

Remember when I mentioned that as you date you get to refine what it is you're looking for? And how when you're fixed on a particular goal—like gathering sexual experience or landing a long-term relationship—while staying open to possibilities, you can create a Dating Zen mindset that's a lot easier to work with than a rigid one? Well, in this chapter, we're going to take an even closer look at exactly how to approach dating with an open mind.

Too often we expect that if we're actively taking steps toward building the life we want, eventually this will pay off in the form of a culminating moment of perfect satisfaction. The flip side to this expectation is that when (not if) we don't get exactly what we're looking for, we think we've done something wrong—that the fault is our own. But the truth is that trying your best will deliver some joy, some pain, some expectations met, some challenges overcome, and others still ahead. Believing that there is a fixed end point to dating can actually hinder your experience of it, and judging yourself for perceived failings will keep you stuck in the belief that you'll never find what you're looking for.

I've seen this in my clients who judge themselves harshly for the way they dated in the past. Their lack of experience, or perception that it took them "so long" to figure out what they want, makes them determined to do dating "right" this time. But experience is gathered bit by bit, and knowledge sometimes comes after we've had many successes and fuck-ups. That's why I always encourage a gentle review of the past and not fixating on the length of time it took to get to this point. Instead, I ask my clients to envision how the experiences they've had so far—even if they've had none—will inform the here and now. We can't know what's going to work for us in advance, and people are far more complex than we can ever understand until we get to know them over time. And that's exactly what dating is! You have to invest time in people to learn about them, and that means that time is never wasted, despite how it might feel.

Approaching dating with this type of judgment can put an undue amount of pressure on yourself and the process. So if you've been carrying around the weight of your dating past, here is some helpful reframing to get unstuck from a negative mindset.

"I'm too old to have as little experience with sex and dating as I do. I'm awful at this!" ➔ "Everyone is trying to gain experience. The goal isn't to be a good dater; it's to find people to connect with and learn from."

"I've wasted a lot of time with people who weren't good for me. There's no one out there for me!" ➜ "There are many types of people I haven't dated yet. I've learned a lot about how I don't want to be treated and know more about what to look out for so I can avoid the kinds of folks I've dated in the past."

"If I haven't found what I'm looking for by now, I doubt anything will happen anytime soon." ➜ "Everyone's timeline is different for finding what they're looking for. I had a future in mind that hasn't come to pass, but that doesn't mean the things I want to happen won't happen eventually for me."

"I've been so hurt in the past, I only know what I don't want." ➜ "Focusing on what I don't want is actually helpful because the inverse of what I don't want is what I *do* want. I can start screening for that now."

Letting go of the judgment you have of your past is a great starting point to staying open to your dating future. Each person we connect with presents opportunities to learn about ourselves and what we truly want. Whether you've been on six hundred dates or none, dating provides a valuable testing ground for figuring out and narrowing down your goals. You'll also learn things about yourself as you engage with different types of people who can bring out sides of you that you may not have experienced before. In this chapter, we'll examine the freedom of being present for whatever life sends your way and how that's never a wasted effort.

HOW TO BE LESS FIXATED ON THE OUTCOME

Have you ever shown up to a date assuming that you know exactly how it will go based on the person you're meeting? Think back to a time when you thought that you had a hookup in your immediate future or that the person was your future co-parent. How did that go? You may have been spot-on and, if so, congratulations! But I wouldn't be surprised if you've had dates that went nowhere near how you were expecting them to go. First dates usually come with a lot of assumptions about the other person based on the limited information we have beforehand. Even if you've had the experience of moving a friendship into romantic territory, there was probably so much you didn't know about what the other person was like sexually or as a romantic partner. Your first real date with this person may have not been anything like what you thought it would be.

Earlier, I encouraged you to ditch your list of must-haves and start focusing on the more qualitative aspects of your initial connections, because it takes time to wrap your head around who someone is and there are always trade-offs. Holding folks to the standard of a checklist limits not only the kinds of people you allow into your dating life but also your expectations of what you think is possible.

My client Audra was someone who found herself rejecting potential partners very early in the dating process because they didn't meet all of her criteria. She just didn't want to waste time on people she didn't think would be good matches. When we started working together, she was exhausted, bewildered, and judging herself for her unfruitful dating past. She wanted more sexual experiences but noticed that the men she was gravitating toward never seemed to put her sexual needs first.

"At this point, I know what I'm gonna get with guys. I just wish I could get some form of intimacy along with my hookups, but is that an oxymoron?" Audra asked.

I told her I didn't think it was unrealistic to want intimacy along with hookups, and then I pivoted our conversation to the guys she had recently rejected. What was the mismatch with each of them? She mentioned that a few of them had zero sense of humor, a couple didn't graduate from college, and one lived at home. These were qualities that were antithetical to her must-have list.

I probed on. "So the guys who you've been having one-night stands with and feeling no intimacy are all college educated with good senses of humor and their own apartments?"

"Well, when you put it that way, I sound like a monster!" she said.

"You're not a monster," I assured her. "I just think you're assuming some pretty major things about guys who haven't shown you much at all, and you're rejecting guys based on other assumptions that may be keeping you from intimacy and better sex."

When I dug deeper into why this might be happening, I learned that Audra was attracted to men who peacock—she saw this as a sign of sexual confidence—and found herself skimming the surface on dates with name-dropping guys who asked her very little about herself. Believing that this might be fine for hookup purposes, she would proceed when they checked most of her must-have boxes. She was now realizing that keeping things surface level meant it was more difficult to get her intimacy needs met. She wanted this to change but was at the point where she believed that this was just how dating was.

We discussed how developing more intimate connections would likely increase the quality of sex she was experiencing, even in a hookup. "But what does that even look like?" she asked.

"Well, for starters, it's being able to feel like you're part of the conversation beforehand." I mentioned that some of my clients have had the hottest sex when they've had discussions with the other person about what each of them likes and doesn't like sexually before meeting up and trying things out. The best part of taking a more sex-positive approach to dating—and expecting the same from your partners—is that you'll both start with a baseline of wanting the experience to be great for everyone involved. You'll also both understand that a little discussion beforehand can go a long way to making that happen. I suggested that Audra do a bit more vetting before committing to in-person dates.

"Assuming that because someone is hot and DTF they're a good sexual match hasn't been working. So what's missing?" I asked.

"I guess more discussion of what I'm about, what I like, and what I'm looking for, which feels scary but could also create the intimacy I'm looking for."

"Great! So after matching and feeling like there's a mutual attraction, can you take the conversation to a flirtatious place and see how they handle you being more forward about what you want?"

After a few attempts to screen out partners who were intimacy averse, Audra was noticing that she had widened her pool of candidates to include people who would not have been on her radar before. They were cuties who didn't check all the boxes on her must-have list, but they were enthusiastic about her desires and seemed really open to seeing where the connection could go.

"Okay, what is happening? I've had a couple really hot hookups recently with guys I actually *like*! It's surprising. This is also very weird timing, because I was just laid off and don't feel great about it. I'm finding some relief in my dating life though. Funny how things happen sometimes." In the end, loosening her grip on what dating and her ideal sexual partners should be like created the space for her to be surprised, even at a time when things weren't perfect in her professional life.

Audra is by no means the only client whose assumptions were limiting their experiences.

Because of his assumptions, Derian struggled with accepting when there was a genuine mismatch. He came to me when he noticed a pattern in his dating life in which things ran their course after a couple months or a handful of dates. Usually the other person broke things off, citing some differences that he had either completely overlooked or didn't believe were deal breakers. A glass-half-full attitude in dating isn't necessarily a bad thing, but it was keeping him from recognizing when things really weren't heading in the right direction.

"It's all so draining," Derian said. "Some of these people I legitimately cared about, and I feel so discarded. It's hard to get back in the game when you think it's just gonna happen again."

I could feel his exhaustion through the phone, so I asked him, "What are you looking to get out of dating right now?"

"Honestly, I'd love to work on having more balance. The high highs and the low lows are maddening, especially with everything else I've got going on in my life. On top of that, I'm ready to settle down. The sooner the better! I want out of the dating pool as soon as possible."

We worked together to tighten up his dating goals and values—he was looking for a partner who shared his faith, wanted a couple kids, and had a shared love of science— as well as ways he could stay present on dates. What was he reading into? What were the facts the other person was sharing about themself? How did he feel when he was with them? After each date that he felt went well, I encouraged him to jot down a few notes about the things that energized him about the person *and* any questions he might have about goals, compatibility, and lifestyles. He collected this data over a couple months and realized that he had never been as present as he was now. He told me he could see how his desire to be off the market made him more likely to just slot someone into the place of "partner" without a lot of analysis of whether he was a good match for them.

Over time, he got better at limiting his tendency to project too far into the future before he got to know the person. Rather than getting carried away by the assumption that this person was "the One" because they got along well, Derian created a more balanced assessment of each person and the dynamic he was building with them over time. As more was revealed, he was better able to factor that into his expectations—and as a result, he developed a couple lovely relationships that he explored simultaneously.

In one of our sessions, he told me that he had decided to cut things off with someone who, he learned, had their heart set on moving back to Europe in a couple years. "Ordinarily I would have just kept seeing them until they boarded the plane and then been miserable afterward. They're a great person and I want to keep in touch, but romantically it's not a good fit, and I know I'll have more energy for dating by backing out now."

I perked up.

"What? Is this progress?" he asked.

"Yes! You've really embraced the process and resisted the urge to force something that didn't feel right for you!" I yelled over our video chat. "You should celebrate."

While Derian was not used to celebrating a breakup, he could recognize that he was breaking a pattern, and that felt like a win.

When you approach dating from the perspective that each new person may teach you more about what you want and don't want, you can trust your experience and ride out the emotional challenges more easily. You might even find the process more enjoyable because, rather than willing yourself through it, you're able to acknowledge what *is* and stress less about what *isn't* happening between you and your dates.

Recognizing your assumptions and trying to challenge them is crucial for approaching relationships with an open mind and not getting too narrowly focused on an expected outcome.

Take a few moments to think about any assumptions you carry into in-person dating.

Do you assume that because someone has a certain job, education, background, or social status that they will behave a certain way, treat you a certain way, or have values similar to yours? What are the characteristics of the people you've been attracted to in the past? Are these characteristics limiting you in any way? Without close inspection, we risk carrying assumptions and stereotypes around that we inherited from our upbringing and culture. This often shows up around race, class, ability, immigrant status, and physical appearance, to name a few. Remember, these might feel like preferences, but when you dig a bit deeper they may indicate a bias that is keeping you from connecting with people who could be better fits for your relationship goals.

We also can fall into a trap of downplaying or overlooking our dates' characteristics that are incompatible with what we're looking for, just because we want to feel like things are progressing. We might see someone as the kind of person we *should* be with, so we choose to look past things that aren't working for us. Just like you can catch yourself when you slip into assumption patterns, you can pause to assess whether what you want feels aligned with what your date has to offer.

EMBRACE PESSIMISM
AND ACKNOWLEDGE YOUR WINS

It's impossible not to bring our preconceived notions about people into dating, but sometimes we're just wrong. We're wrong about how attracted we'll be to them, what kind of person they are, how attentive they'll be to us, and on and on. There's nothing wrong with being wrong—both when the truth is better than what we expected and when it's worse. Either way, we gain more information than we had before the date. Keeping an open mind means that you're just as willing to connect with someone as you are to not connect if it's in your best interest. Because the fact is, you won't like everyone and not everyone will like you.

There are too many unknowns in the beginning stages of dating to get caught up in being right about someone. It's actually a setup for disappointment and can put a huge damper on your energy.

Take my client Jia. They were so down on themself each time a person wasn't a match that they believed they had terrible instincts and would be perpetually single.

"I guess I'm just really pessimistic," they said.

"Believing you're never going to find someone is fatalistic, not pessimistic. A healthy dose of pessimism can actually be really helpful when dating!* Being pessimistic means that you don't expect things or people to be perfect and that

---

* The School of Life, "How to Make Love Last," virtual class, School of Life, accessed on July 6, 2020, www.theschooloflife.com/events /how-to-make-love-last.

you anticipate some amount of disappointment." I then went on to explain how pessimism can buffer you from unrealistic expectations and can help make the process smoother and more fun.

There's no such thing as the perfect match, but there are plenty of "good enough" matches that come with their own unique challenges. Think about it: the world is too big for you to not find folks with whom you'll connect. Whether you're looking for a relationship, sex, or both, other people are looking for something similar. You just have to find each other and stay open to what less-than-ideal qualities you each inevitably will have. Every single person, including us, has some imperfect qualities. The trick is finding matches with comparable or compatible flaws.*

If this is all hitting you too hard, I get it. We receive a lot of messages about partnership that conflict with this idea. Soul mates and "You complete me" and true-love narratives dominate the way we talk about partnership. Not to mention that finding this elusive perfect person is supposed to be easy ("When you know, you know"), but also somehow hard ("Relationships are hard work"), and so worth it ("You can have it all if you just try harder!"). So often we're told not to settle, but every relationship dynamic involves settling to some degree. This isn't necessarily a bad thing, though. There are many instances when people settle in the interest of getting an approximation of what they want, and it's not seen as

---

*Alain de Botton, "Why You Will Marry the Wrong Person," *New York Times*, May 28, 2016, www.nytimes.com/2016/05/29/opinion/sunday/why-you-will-marry-the-wrong-person.html.

a terrible thing. In fact, in pretty much every other aspect of our lives besides dating, it's expected that we compromise or accept conditions that are less than perfect. We don't always get the job we want with the pay we need, or if we do, there may be aspects of the job that we hate. Our relationships with friends require a certain amount of settling, as we can't control when our friends decide to move and we can't pick their partners for them—we have to accept the fact that their choices aren't ours. But somehow, in sex and dating we are expected to settle for nothing less than perfection.

Being a little pessimistic about your dating life doesn't mean you stop looking for people with whom you feel really good. It just means looking at dating as you would any other aspect of life. You will make choices that you think are good in the moment, evaluate how those choices work for you, and then make new choices based on what you've learned. The more you can accept that dating is an imperfect process—and let go of the impossible standards that society has placed on it—the easier it will become. And the easier it is, the happier you will be in the long run with your choices.

Being pessimistic doesn't mean being sad and negative all the time either. Expecting that things won't always be great means that you can better recognize when they are. In fact, your definition of success might even open up, giving you *more* to celebrate. One of the ways you can help keep yourself from experiencing dating burnout is to celebrate any wins you experience, big or small. If you leave a first date feeling relatively good, that's a win. If you leave feeling like you just dodged a bullet, that's a win. If you get a second date you wanted, that's a win. And if someone rejects you before the second date, that's also a win because you are released from thinking that this person is a viable option. When you decide to start dating, celebrate yourself for even trying!

Now take a moment to think of five things you can celebrate. They don't have to be major accomplishments or even super positive. They could be anything from reading this book to hooking up with someone for the first time to being dumped. Celebrating the good, the bad, and the ugly of dating allows you to stay grounded for whatever comes your way. It's a great way to truly embrace the process.

AVOID BIGGER BETTER DEAL SYNDROME

When you combine the belief that you can have it all with the access to hundreds, sometimes thousands, of people that dating apps provide, you create favorable conditions for Bigger Better Deal Syndrome to emerge. This is when you pass up strong connections because you think that there is someone else who could make you happier or who's more attractive or better off financially or more of whatever other markers of compatibility you may have. Believing that there's someone better than the person you're seeing or hooking up with seriously devalues that person and everything they bring to the experience. If no one is perfect, including you, then the pursuit of a perfect match is a futile quest. So why do so many people embark upon it?

I see BBDS in my clients all the time. Making too many assumptions about people and faultfinding tends to make my clients not only burn out but also feel generally miserable. Often, I see BBDS in folks who fear being judged themselves.

They employ a tactic of "reject first" to avoid the deeper connection that comes with being vulnerable and exposing all the imperfections that make them who they are.

Mira was a client like this. She had had a string of relationships that ended when she found out, to her surprise, that her partners had flaws. Why was the universe doing this to her? She had a good heart and so much to give to "the right person." When I asked her who this right person was, she explained that it would be someone who totally got her and loved everything about who she was and what she wanted in life. She had her list, yes, but there were also intangibles that she desired as well. She believed that the right person and she would have immediate, undeniable chemistry, share all of the same pastimes, have a similar cultural background and political ideology, make about the same amount of money, have similar travel styles, and be fluent in the same languages. The person she felt came closest to this wasn't as physically attractive to her as some of her other partners. She had tried to make it work but couldn't get past the fact that, while she was attracted to her partner, they just weren't the hottest. She felt that if she could get this close to perfection, why stop there?

You might identify with Mira or you may have been in a relationship with someone who was busy comparing you to what they had or could have with other people. Either position is brutal. The BBDS sufferer misses out on getting to know and connecting with someone who is a pretty good match. And the person on the other side is subjected to the pain of feeling not good enough. Nobody wins.

If you catch yourself slipping into BBDS, it may be a sign that you should take a break from dating and consider what you are truly looking for. Think about how you can shift your dating strategy away from mining for gold to collecting gems along the way. It's also worth considering how you would feel with the same high standards applied to you and if maybe you are pushing away great people to keep yourself from being judged for your flaws.

HOW TO STAY GROUNDED AND FOCUSED WHEN EMOTIONS ARE HIGH

Dating can be a rocky, emotional journey as people who stir up feelings ranging from excitement and desire to revulsion and disappointment are thrown into your path. That can make staying grounded while dating pretty difficult. If you get swept up in how spectacularly poorly a date went, it makes it hard to move forward. Likewise, if you make a strong connection and aren't grounded in reality from time to time, you could get distracted by a less-than-stellar match.

The good news is that getting back to solid ground is a skill you can improve with practice. Below are some examples of things you can do to keep yourself steady or get back on track after an emotional blow.

- Keep a dating journal. After each high high or low low, give yourself some time to write out what happened and how it made you feel. Over time, you may see helpful patterns about what kinds of dates and people felt the best and what really doesn't work for you.

- Take five deep, clearing breaths when you feel over-whelmed by an emotion. This can help bring you back into the present moment, which is hopefully more pleasant.

- Get physical. When emotions are high, it can be hard to think clearly, and that limits our ability to assess what is truly happening in our dating lives. Move-ment of any kind can help get us out of our heads and allow us to process what happened through our bodies. Take a walk, do twenty jumping jacks, hug a friend, dance, spin around in circles, or do an exer-cise of your choice.

- Debrief with a friend or therapist. You might occa-sionally vent to a friend when things get rough, and when things are really hard it could be good to pro-cess your emotions with a trained therapist or other mental-health provider.

EXERCISE: PREPARING FOR DATES WITH AN OPEN MIND

Every date has the possibility of connection, rejection, or honestly just being meh. It's okay to feel let down if someone seems awesome at first and then doesn't deliver in person. It's also good to remember not to lean too heavily on an out-come *before* the date even happens. Keep in mind just how nerve-racking first dates can be. Your date may be too anx-ious or afraid to be their true self right away.

Before a date, try this thought experiment: Think of the time you will spend with your date as being full of possibilities. Allow yourself to think of a few outcomes and let yourself feel all of the feelings that might come with those outcomes. You can fantasize about going home with them and having amazing sex, or you can imagine them spilling their food all over you and ruining your favorite item of clothing. Just let yourself imagine what the date might hold—good, bad, and neutral.

When you've run through a few scenarios, tell yourself that literally anything is possible and that, in most cases, you will be just fine, whether the date is a raging success or utter disaster. This is the truth, so take a moment to really feel it.

A lot of our enjoyment in life comes from being pleasantly surprised by situations and outcomes. Having assumptions about how things will go before you even meet someone could seriously diminish the possibility of being pleasantly surprised. Be open. From this position, you don't have to give up completely if something you were expecting doesn't happen. Being open to possibility is a courtesy that most people want but find difficult to give to others, so try it—release yourself and your date from unhelpful assumptions that get in the way of your experience. When you keep an open mind, there is absolutely no need for a checklist of things you want from the other person. Instead, the connection becomes the focus.

PART 3
LEAVE IT BETTER THAN YOU FOUND IT

9

Date One and Done

We must accept finite disappointment,
but never lose infinite hope.

—MARTIN LUTHER KING JR.

We've all been there: the first-date fizzle. They were so good on paper, and so bad for us in person. Most of the time these mismatches are good humans; we just didn't feel a connection with them. If you think this happens to you a lot, you're not alone. In fact, the first-date fizzle is one of the biggest (and most common) disappointments in dating, because after all of the hard work you did to weed out bad matches and find common ground with someone you're attracted to, there can still be a disconnect.

Sometimes this disconnect is circumstantial. One of you isn't feeling great and, rather than cancel, shows up to the date unavailable for what the experience could be. This type of disconnect can be something you come back from by chatting after the date, clarifying what happened, and seeing if another date goes better. But sometimes the disconnect is unavoidable—your conversational rhythm is off and it's not because of nerves. You really don't share a sense of humor, or your values don't align. Sometimes people do a much better job at connecting via text or DM and aren't able to replicate that in person. This is hard stuff, and it can be incredibly frustrating because until you meet the person face-to-face, you won't know that it's a bad match.

There's a lot to take in on that first in-person date. Although the goal is to stay open to possibilities, you also have to absorb as much information as you can so you can decide whether you want to see this person again. You may not be able to process everything while you're on the date, and that's fine. Your date will hopefully be doing the same kind of processing, which is why sometimes you may feel that a date ended really well but then the other person lets you know that they didn't feel the same. There are so many reasons why first dates go nowhere. There can be the obvious rejection of the match by either or both parties. But there can also be more subtle, behind-the-scenes issues, ranging from how you compare to other people the person is dating to how each of you smells, talks, kisses, has sex, etc.

So what should you do if you're not vibing with your date, despite all your efforts? This chapter will provide guidance on how to set each date up for your maximum enjoyment, regardless of how the connection goes. We'll also get into how to exit dud dates gracefully and deliver rejections with kindness. Because let's face it, all of us will experience rejection at some point, so we could stand to get better at both giving and receiving it.

GETTING COMFORTABLE ON DATES

Staying open on dates does not mean subjecting yourself to unpleasantness. Your comfort matters! So often I see folks have agreed to dates that aren't ideal for them, but because the other person seemed excited about it, they went along and subsequently had an awful time. First dates often need a bit of planning and discussion to set both parties up for success. Letting your date know that what they've suggested isn't ideal, for whatever reason, is part of giving the first date a fair shot. Sometimes, if the conditions aren't great, it's hard to get comfortable and assess your connection accurately.

This was certainly the case for my client Suni. Recently sober, she was finding it difficult to reject bar dates but struggled to advocate for her comfort.

"It's not that I'm worried that I'll drink. It's more that I feel like I'm over that whole bar scene. I'm kinda turned off by the drunken party vibe now," she said.

"I hear you. Bars aren't always the best place to assess chemistry—they can be distracting and irritating if you're not into it. Also, does insisting on a less boozy atmosphere make you feel like you have to discuss your sobriety right away?" I asked.

"Yeah, sometimes. It's not something I'm ashamed of so much as it feels unsexy to discuss right at the beginning," she explained. "When I'm able to set the date up, I usually choose a non-bar place that serves alcohol. But when someone wants to meet up for a late-night hang, it feels like the easiest thing is just to go to a bar, and then I'm that person having to explain why I'm ordering a soda at ten p.m. It's awkward."

Suni was struggling with the common expectation that bars are a natural first-date spot and how that environment made her less comfortable on dates. Sometimes, she confessed, her annoyance with being in a bar was so great that she actually moved dates to her house or the other person's quicker than she ordinarily would.

"So this is really impacting your sex life?" I asked.

"Yeah, and not in a super great way. Those hookups tended to be fine but not amazing. I wish I could have eased into things a bit more," she said. We then discussed places where Suni could steer dates who wanted to meet up for a late-night drink that weren't bars and talked about ways she could reveal her sobriety on her own terms.

"There's this supercute diner near me that's open late. It's got a kitschy vibe that's very me, and they also have a liquor license. It can be a bit of a scene, but I don't feel nearly as agitated as I do in straight-up bars when I'm there." This became Suni's go-to spot for dates when she planned them or if the person suggested a bar meetup. Was every date great? No. But she was noticing how that small change of venue really supported her being fully present no matter what.

Another client, Jayla, shared with me that she stopped going on dates anywhere there was a large crowd because it activated not only her anxiety but also her stutter. This compounded her first-date jitters and made it hard for her to relax. Some of my clients apply a boundary around going to someone else's house or apartment to hook up. They prefer hosting, at least at first, because they are literally more at home in their own environment. Others feel more comfortable with their hookups not knowing where they live, so they make their place off-limits until they know the person more.

Putting your comfort front and center gives you more freedom on the date and can set you up for a more pleasurable experience. The idea is to limit the ways you might be unnecessarily distracted or overwhelmed in an already stressful situation. Of course, your date will have needs too, but it's good to think about what your ideal date conditions might be so you can have them in mind as you plan together.

Take a few moments to think about the conditions that make you feel the most comfortable when you are out in the world in general. This may include types of places where you feel at ease, events you enjoy attending, or times of the day or week when you have the most energy to be social. Write your thoughts below.

I feel most comfortable when I'm _____

_____

Places where I feel most like myself include _____

_____

When getting to know someone, I appreciate an atmosphere of _____

_____

Advocating for your ideal conditions can help you feel your best on dates, no matter what happens. Yes, you will probably be a little nervous and maybe a bit uncomfortable at first—that part is natural—but at least you'll know that you collaborated with your date to try to make the experience mutually enjoyable, regardless of the outcome between you.

Below are some general suggestions to ensure a safer, more comfortable first date. If, within these parameters, someone makes you feel unsafe, or like the date is going nowhere, you can exit knowing you did everything you could to make it fun.

1. Suggest a public place to meet first. Spending time with someone in a public setting allows both of you to settle in and get comfortable. If all goes well, you can discuss whether you would like to move the date to a private spot later (even on that same date), but it's good to have that public buffer at first so you can see if there's a connection that feels worth exploring.

2. Choose places where you feel particularly comfortable. Feeling comfortable means a lot of things and can encompass physical, emotional, and financial well-being. During early COVID, a lot of my clients opted for socially distanced outdoor dates with masks. Asking for this before the date meant that the other person was aware of their comfort level with in-person contact and could act accordingly or opt out if they disagreed. If you have a disability that needs accommodating, you may be more aware of certain spaces' accessibility limitations. You can suggest places that you know you'll

be able to access safely and comfortably. If the person suggests an expensive restaurant or event without explicitly stating that it will be their treat, and you aren't comfortable spending that amount of money, you can suggest another option that's within your financial reach. You don't need to say *why* you prefer a certain place, just that you would like to meet there instead of where the other person suggested.

3. Stay open to the comfort needs of others. If someone has a concern about when, where, and how the date takes place, hear them out and see if you can find a compromise between your needs and theirs. For instance, insisting that a person come across town to your neighborhood might not work for them given their schedule and energy. Be open to meeting halfway if that helps cut down their commute.

So what if all of your needs are met, but you're still uncomfortable for whatever reason? It's okay to tell the other person what you need, whether that's moving the date to another environment that's more comfortable for you or telling them that their line of questioning makes you uncomfortable, or even that you would prefer they not touch you until you've had more time to get to know them. Sometimes saying what you need is all it takes for the other person to make adjustments or apologize. And sometimes, you just have to bolt.

WHEN TO STAY AND
WHEN TO CALL IT A NIGHT

Taking steps to ensure that you're going to be as comfortable on a date as you can be is great, but we all know that the best-laid plans often go awry. If someone makes you feel uncomfortable by the way they are talking to or about you or if they are crossing any personal boundaries, you are entirely permitted to leave without much of an explanation. A simple "I have to go" is enough.

So many people stay on dates that are truly going nowhere out of politeness. I'm here to tell you that you can be polite *and* spare yourself the agony of sitting through hours of bad conversation or worse. Sometimes politeness really isn't required, especially if someone has been rude to you.

If you're anything like my client Davey, you may want to set a time limit for first dates. Davey employed a one-hour rule. That meant that if after one hour they weren't enjoying themselves, they would explain that they were meeting a friend (which was often true) or they needed to have an early night before a tough day ahead (again, often true). If the date was going well, they would consider whether they wanted to stay or quit while they were ahead. On occasion, Davey would leave a date before an hour had passed. In these rare instances, the other person was a jerk by their estimation. Davey had already gotten accustomed to cutting dates short, so they just pulled the rip cord early and found ways to salvage their night like treating themself to dinner or blowing off steam with a friend.

Having a time limit—an hour or whatever feels good to you—is a great way to keep a first meeting super casual while you get a feel for who the other person is. It's a brilliant strategy for managing your energy.

Sometimes it's hard to be the person to leave a date, even if you have clear reasons to do so. It's even harder when you're not sure whether the person is terrible or just a giant ball of nerves. Below is a chart to help determine whether your date is nervous or is actually being a jerk. Notice there is some overlap, so a good rule of thumb is that if your date does any of the actions in the second column and is making you regret you came, or if they exhibit a few of these bad behaviors, feel free to leave!

Signs a Person May Be Nervous	Signs a Person May Be an Ass
Overly chatty, doesn't give you space to talk	Overly chatty, doesn't give you space to talk
Shy or reserved, hard to open up	Doesn't ask you anything about yourself
Overly apologetic	Doesn't apologize
Unsure of where to take the conversation	Rude to anyone, including server/bartender
Won't stop looking at their phone	Won't stop looking at their phone
Sweaty, flushed, or jittery	Makes inappropriate gestures or comments about your body
Makes a poorly timed or awkward joke	Makes a joke at your expense, says you're too sensitive if you react

These are just a few common signs, and you may have your own list of indicators of a date's nerves or ass-ness. Recognizing these signals will help you decide whether it's a good idea to leave or not.

If you decide to come up with your own time limit for dates, that's great! But when your time is up, how will you know if it's going well?

Ava struggled with knowing when to stay or leave dates so much that she was ready to quit dating altogether. She second-guessed whether she was actually having a good time. "I think I might give the wrong people a second chance and totally give up on people I might actually like. How the hell am I supposed to know the difference?!"

I empathized with Ava's dilemma. There are so many conflicting messages about what a first date should feel like and a lot of unhelpful, unrealistic advice out there about what makes someone a good match. Ava was feeling a tremendous amount of pressure to make the "right choice" about her dates, sometimes going against her better judgment.

It's easy to get caught up in our hopes and dreams for a date and forget that the main goal of dating is to learn about others and ourselves. That means that we may fall back on old ideas about the kinds of people we should want instead of checking in with ourselves about how we actually feel.

Below are some common reasons to stay on a first date or pursue a second date.

- You had fun! Regardless of what you did on the date, you enjoyed yourself and that's enough reason to want more.

- The sexual chemistry is intriguing. Some people are a joy to our senses. Mutual attraction can sometimes be hard to come by, so when it comes, explore it.

- You feel at home. Sometimes the connection is so easy from the beginning that a first date actually feels more like reuniting with an old friend.

- You have really strong common ground. Some folks just get you because of a common background, specific shared interests, or cultural references. This isn't always the case, so be sure to give this rarity a fair shot.

TO GHOST OR NOT TO GHOST?

Ah, ghosting. It has become expected as part of the dating process—you date, therefore you ghost. I'd like this to change. And guess what? That change starts with you. Be the change you want to see in dating! Stop ghosting people, and they will (hopefully) stop ghosting you.

Ghosting has existed in one form or another since humans created courtship rituals. Simply put, it's cutting off all communication after connecting with someone, and it can happen at any stage of dating. People ghost after matching, chatting, the first date, the first time they have sex, a few dates, becoming an official couple, and even, sadly, after years of dating. With the many modes of communication we now use—texting, DMing, phone calls, video chat, email, and so on—ghosting feels particularly harsh. At least in the past if you didn't get a response to your written letter, you could allow yourself to believe it got lost in the mail! Now there's no way to unknow that you've been ghosted across multiple platforms.

Most daters that I have worked with have been ghosted at some point and have even dabbled in ghosting others. It can feel like a hard habit to break when you know that everyone else is doing it too. But I've coached folks through the awkwardness of breaking things off more directly, and I can safely say that, while it seems like more work, it is usually the best option (unless the other person was an ass). Most of the time, the person on the receiving end of an explanation for why someone doesn't want to see them again is super appreciative of this non-ghost-like behavior. It's like a breath of fresh air in a dating world full of dusty ghosts.

Take my client Bahar, who was a self-proclaimed ghoster before we worked together. She had no problem getting dates and enjoyed the process of meeting lots of new people, hooking up, and moving on. The problem she struggled with most was communication, and that was showing up in lots of ways in her sex life. To start, she hadn't been able to have orgasms with partners and found that she deferred to their needs over her own. She always had orgasms through masturbation, so she was confused by the lack of them in partnered sex. I asked if she had ever shared this with the people she was hooking up with. "God no! I just keep hoping someone will come along who knows what to do!" she said.

Bahar ghosted people who disappointed her sexually and with whom she didn't want to have an awkward conversation about her own pleasure. This is actually really common among my clients. A lot of folks feel that if a sexual connection isn't great the first time, it's not worth the trouble pursuing. The reality is that a lot of first-time hookups need tweaking to make them truly enjoyable for everyone involved.

While orgasm isn't a universal measure of enjoyment, it's inaccessibility in Bahar's hookups led us to work on her overall communication skills. We started with her reaching out to her most recent ghosting haunt, someone whom she had slept with a couple weeks prior and whom she had left on read when he reached out to schedule another meetup.

"In a perfect world, what would you say to this person?" I asked.

"That I'm not that into him and I thought the sex would be better."

"Okay, great. We can work with that! Are you totally not into him or are you not into him because the sex was so bad?"

"More the latter."

"So you might want to see him again, just not in a sexual capacity?"

"I guess. We actually clicked really well before we hooked up."

She came up with the following response: "Hey, sorry it has taken me a minute to get back to you. I've had a hard time reaching out because I feel more of a friend vibe between us and I think things got weird after we hooked up. I'm working on being a better communicator and I hope we can hang in the future." I told her to send this text, walk away from her phone, and do something distracting for a while in case it took him some time to get back to her.

In another session, Bahar shared that the guy had responded pretty quickly that he understood where she was coming from. He even seemed excited about hanging out as friends. He reminded her that he was new in town and could use more friends to help him get adjusted to the city. His response was not only shocking for Bahar but also validating that she could be more open about what she was thinking and feeling throughout the dating process. While it was nerve-racking to figure out what she wanted to say and go through with sending the text, she said that it actually left her feeling better than ghosting had. It also made her believe that she should try giving sexual feedback to future partners and see if that improved her experiences.

WHAT'S WITH BREADCRUMBING?

Breadcrumbing is the phenomenon of showing interest in someone—in virtual spaces primarily, but it can extend to in-person interactions as well—without much follow-through. It's like leaving little crumbs of affection for someone to nibble, but it's never enough to fill up on. These gestures take the form of following you on social media, liking posts, sending heart emojis in response to your stories, sending an occasional text, and maybe even flirting with you outright. The moment you try to make something happen with the breadcrumber, however, they vanish or back off their displays of interest for a while. They are evasive, confusing, and downright frustrating in their inconsistent behavior.

Some people think of breadcrumbing as leading someone on, and it can be. People often breadcrumb when they are talking to a few people at a time or if they've started seeing someone but aren't completely ready to go all-in on one person. Being on the receiving end of this type of behavior is maddening until you recognize it for what it is: flattery. It's flattering when someone you find interesting shows interest in you too. But it is dating folly to pursue a breadcrumber in earnest. When someone is truly interested in you, they will make an effort to spend time with you. So if you have tried to hang out with a cutie and they disappear afterward, file this under breadcrumbing and move on. If their situation changes, they may resurface, but it's safe to leave the next move to them.

If you are guilty of breadcrumbing, think about what's behind your small signs of affection. Are you really interested in making something happen with the other person? Can you make a bolder gesture, or do you have circumstances that limit how you can engage, such as your relationship status, location, emotional availability, or fear of rejection? There's meaning behind your actions that can help you understand your own dating needs. Those breadcrumbs aren't just for the other person! Perhaps you are someone who, regardless of relationship status, needs to feel free to flirt. This might point to something you can address with current or future partners.

ACCEPTING REJECTION

One of the hardest parts of dating is enduring rejection. It sucks no matter how or when it happens. But you've done so much work to find your best matches already and, believe it or not, feeling rejection is part of doing just that. When someone rejects you, it is their way of letting you know that the two of you aren't a good match. You aren't the only person who gets to decide, so they are actually helping you make the best decision for you. Rejection can be difficult to reframe, because so often it doesn't feel helpful—it feels shitty.

But it's best to depersonalize rejection, even when it's hard not to see it as deeply personal.

The reality is that rejection disproportionately affects some folks. All of the isms and biases that affect people in their daily lives can also rear their ugly heads in dating. A lot of my clients are people of color who experience rejection throughout the dating process, from matching to in-person dates. Others are fat and feel rejected before they even get a chance to show who they are. Many of my clients have chronic mental or physical health concerns that, once revealed, may make them seem less desirable to certain people. And for my clients with disabilities, finding partners who can fully see them, and not just their disability, is a minefield of rejection.

Feeling like you have limited choices based on how the world sees you is also a form of rejection. It can be liberating to know that the people who are left are there for you and everything that being you means, but I don't expect everyone to experience the shift from rejected to liberated right away. Some of my clients face huge and taxing challenges just trying to find folks who will fully accept them. So much so that I don't expect those feelings of rejection to dissipate even when they find good matches. Most of my clients of color, particularly Black women, enter dating with assumptions that they won't get what they want from the experience and don't deserve to have too many expectations. They have a hard time putting their truths out there because of past experiences of being overlooked or underrated. We have a lot of conversations about what it would feel like to ask for more, be accepted fully, and be seen as desirable. Getting to a place of feeling like that's even possible might take longer for them than for some of my other clients who haven't had to grapple with rejection on such a systemic level.

My client Alexa pushed herself to be visible in ways she had never been comfortable with before. She avoided showing her whole body in profile pictures because of her weight. Her general resistance to setting up a dating profile and showing herself fully came from a deep fear of rejection and the pain she still carried from previous rejections. We worked closely and slowly to make sure that she could open up on her own time, so it was to my surprise when she shared that she had added a swimsuit photo to her dating profile. Showing her body to anyone—let alone strangers on the internet—was incredibly vulnerable, but, she explained, "I can't deny how utterly happy I look in this photo. And I felt magnetic the day it was taken. That's how I want to be seen and that's what I want people to want."

What followed was not a series of rejections but rather an outpouring of adoration and admiration from potential matches. For someone who always felt too big to be pretty, and who had been seen as cute rather than sexy, she was now in awe of herself. She was also seeing rejection in a whole new way. "These men are showing up for me in ways that others in my past never did. And when I have sex, I'm more in my body because I know they see and want me. I can't fucking believe it."

Each of my clients faces rejection at some point in the dating process. We work together when this happens to reframe it as something that does not determine their worth but instead leads them to more fulfilling connections. The belief that rejection, though often painful, brings them closer to their dating and relationship goals is what sustains them.

Remarkably, rejection is something that, over time, we can all get better at accepting and reconciling with the unique factors that make us who we are. The rejections along the way can help make getting what we want in the end that much sweeter.

How has rejection impacted your dating experience?

How might you release a bit of the pain, frustration, and fear that rejection stirs in you? How can you begin to accept rejection as a necessary part of getting to experience the connections you really want?

EXERCISE: REJECTING WITH KINDNESS

When it's clear that someone isn't for you, it's tempting to just disappear, but we could all do with a little more kindness in the world. Breaking things off directly isn't easy, but it's a good way to work on your dating karma. To make the process less daunting, it's a good idea to have a few responses ready for when the temptation to ghost flares up.

Examples include:

- *Thanks so much for last night. It was great meeting you, but I don't think we're looking for the same things. I hope you find what you're looking for.*

- *I'm glad we got to meet up! You're great, but I just didn't feel a romantic/sexual connection.*

- *Thanks for coming out last night! I've had fun getting to know you and think I see this as more of a friendship. I hope you're open to that.*

Use the examples above or craft a couple of your own responses that will help you be clear and kind when it's your turn to deliver rejection.

Dating involves assessing how well things are progressing over time, and not everyone will agree. Sometimes dates flop big-time. Sometimes we are rejected outright before we feel we have the chance to show who we are, or we have to reject someone based on how we feel with them. Regardless of which side you're on, rejection is never easy. I hope you resist the urge to ghost and that you communicate what's not working for you. And I encourage you to shift away from the notion that rejections are a reflection of how worthy you are as a dater. Everyone deserves to find connections that work for them, and rejections are just one hurdle to jump over on the way to your goals.

10

When I Get That Feeling,
I Need Sexual Feedback

The ability to critique oneself and change and
to hear critique from others is the condition of
being that makes us capable of responsibility.

—BELL HOOKS

Whether we acknowledge it or not, we all carry some responsibility as we date. Our actions have consequences, and we're responsible for how we treat ourselves and others. We're also responsible for breaking some really powerful taboos that keep us from having better, more connected experiences sexually and non-sexually with others. If we want the culture of dating to truly change—to be as fun as possible for as many people as possible—we have to break the taboo around talking about sex.

When you make connections that you feel good about, moving those connections into sexual territory is super common. But folks get nervous when they have to communicate their sexual desires and needs. Doing so is one of the ways that you can maximize your enjoyment of dating or continue to grow within a new relationship. And being able to receive the desires and needs of others and act in ways that affirm them is a great way to be a better partner.

We've discussed how communicating your needs through-out dating is a skill that most of us have to develop with prac-tice. That means we may get it wrong a few times along the way. We may also struggle with knowing exactly what we want to communicate from time to time, and that's okay. A particular place where I see this come up is in sexual commu-nication. One person wants something the other doesn't, or one person wants something to be different but they may not know exactly how to make it better. One person may try in their own way to redirect the other person, but for whatever reason the attempt is lost in sexual translation. The conse-quence of this lack of clear and open communication ranges from meh sex to terrible sex.

Sexual feedback is next-level communication. It requires us to be vulnerable while holding firm to our ideals about how we want sex to be. There comes a time in everyone's life when they have to speak up on behalf of their own sexual enjoyment, and I want you to feel confident doing so sooner rather than later. I want you to become comfortable with the idea that great sex doesn't always just happen and recognize that you actually have a lot of communication tools at your disposal—you may just need practice using them.

If the thought of giving sexual feedback feels scary, that's because most of us have had little to no guidance on exactly how to communicate sexually. When you think back to your experience in sex-education class (if you had one) there was probably no discussion about how to communicate with partners about what you like and the types of sexual experiences you're looking for. Most of us received sex education that focused on reproduction and how to avoid pregnancy and STIs. Not only is that stuff not applicable to a lot of types of sex, but it completely overlooks pleasure. That's why it's not surprising when clients tell me that they don't know what they want sexually, aren't sure how to ask for it if they do, and are terrified of giving feedback in bed. A lot of their fears are based on either negative experiences they've had as a result of speaking up or the belief that a perfect partner would innately know what they want and do it without any guidance.

There is no way to feel confident in any subject when you are ill-prepared, and most of us are ill-prepared when it comes to sexual communication. That means that there are a lot of unconfident people doing the best they can with what they've got. Lack of education, unclear and even iffy sexual experiences, and information that overgeneralizes what it means to have good sex all work together to create the perfect storm of sexual disempowerment.

The trick to delivering sexual feedback with confidence is to remember the following:

1. You probably haven't been given much information or encouragement about talking about sexual desires, and neither has anyone else. We're all in this together, and we need to give each other space to figure things out.

2. No one else has knowledge of your body like you do. Getting intimately acquainted with what you like

and how you like it is the best way to give yourself more language for when feedback is needed.

3. Every single person's sexuality is unique, including yours! To assume that anyone else is going to like sex in the exact same way as you or your previous partners is setting an unrealistic expectation. Not everyone will be an ideal sexual match for you, but communication can sometimes help bridge the gap between your differences.

4. You can be your own advocate. If you experience discomfort or pain or are generally not into what is going on sexually, you have the right to express this, suggest other activities, or stop completely.

With the above in mind, I urge you to take a more curious and generous approach to sex, especially sex with new partners. That's when sex can be the most fun—when you're learning each other and hopefully working really hard to make the most of each sexual experience you have together. Know that even with the best chemistry things can and will go awry, but that doesn't mean that you have to have terrible sex in silence. In this chapter, I'll explain how to give feedback that transforms awkward moments or sexual misalignments into sex that truly delivers the pleasure you deserve.

Let's start with a visualization exercise.

Imagine yourself a couple years in the future. You have some sexual experiences under your belt—some good, some bad. But as you are standing in your future life, you know that you are clearer and more confident about what you want from sex. You recognize that the moments when you pushed through to communicate your sexual needs actually led to better experiences, or at least more information about your sexual compatibility with others. You were also on the receiving end of some feedback about how you are sexually. Some of it you agree with, and some of it you chalk up to a difference in your sexual desires. In short, you've learned how to be a better sexual communicator and partner.

Take a few breaths to really sink into this future you, and read on for the steps you can take to become that version of yourself.

HOW TO ADDRESS A SEXUAL MISALIGNMENT

Remember those sexual values you discovered in Chapter 2? This is when you really get to claim them. Hopefully you have been supporting yourself sexually throughout dating by using your masturbation practice, maybe even taking notes about what you like and don't like. Your values and self-knowledge form the basis for the language you can use when you need to give a partner some oh-so-valuable sexual feedback.

Many of my clients become pros at sexual feedback, bringing all of their self-knowledge to their sexual encounters. Like my client Charlie, who started out feeling uncomfortable during sex and had a hard time talking about why. Her early experiences with dating were defined by her trying to emulate how she thought the other person wanted her to be during sex. That meant that there were a lot of faked orgasms and a lack of genuine pleasure on her part. She recognized that there was a big disconnect between her experiences with self-pleasure, where she always orgasmed, and partnered sex. When she learned to center her values of playfulness, challenge, and seduction and focus her partners on the kinds of stimulation she needed, she found that she enjoyed herself more.

Her breakthrough happened on a date with someone she had been seeing for a while. They had hooked up a few times and she had never orgasmed. She insisted on being on top that night, a position that she knew would give her more clitoral stimulation. When he made a move to switch positions, she teased him, saying, "What, you can't handle how good this feels? I think this is exactly what you need because it's exactly what I need." He told her that what she was doing felt amazing and that he wanted whatever she wanted. It was the first time she felt sexually empowered.

Similarly, my client Carl, who had some specific ways he knew he could orgasm, felt embarrassed to share this with partners. A few of his sexual values included authenticity, respect, and stability, so he decided to focus on finding a partner with whom he could feel comfortable enough to be his full authentic self. He recognized that having a more stable partner, even though they hadn't defined the relationship, gave him a lot more comfort when it came to talking about his needs. So instead of making a polite excuse and downplaying his own desires, he spoke up and shared his technique for orgasming.

"I need a lot of pressure on my cock while my balls are held. Can you try that this time?" he asked. To his delight, this partner heard him and made it their mission to deliver the kind of stimulation he needed. It took a few conversations and adjustments to get things just right, but it was excellent practice for him to give sexual feedback.

Another client, Denise, was recently divorced and realized that she had not had to describe what she liked to anyone in over fifteen years! She spent some time thinking about her previous sex life, what she enjoyed and what she had always wanted but couldn't achieve with her ex. Newly single, she was also dating across the gender spectrum for the first time. When she started a new sexual relationship, she shared her values of adventure, curiosity, and growth, putting herself in a position of being open to possibilities. She found that with these partners she was able to explore her sexual edges and learn so much about how she can connect with different bodies and desires. Her sexual feedback sometimes came in the form of admitting that she was new to certain things and that she needed guidance. To her surprise, many of her partners were open and willing to show her the ropes—sometimes literally, as with one partner who wanted to be tied up and showed Denise how to do it safely.

Knowing your values, what you like, and what you'd like to explore are great first steps to being a better sexual communicator. You can straight up tell or show someone how you do things and what works for your body. And if you're not sure how partnered sex will go because you are out of practice or new to sex, you can let your partner know that you're figuring things out and that you may have lots of feedback along the way as you learn.

A big part of effective sexual communication is feeling like your partner is open to and available for your pleasure. You cannot express yourself freely with someone who shuts you down when you make suggestions, ask for modifications, or share your preferences. These folks are likely to dismiss any feedback you give and cross the boundaries that you share with them. The sexual communication advice I share in the pages that follow is meant to be used with partners who have shown that they are invested in mutually pleasurable, cocreated sexual experiences with you. Throughout, I will provide a few notes about when you might show extra caution. But in general, the ideas that follow are meant to support you with people who you feel will want you to have the best time possible and who know that they have to be open to feedback for that to happen.

If you ever feel unsafe communicating your needs, you may need to leave a sexual situation. Please know that sexual communication also includes reporting any negative experiences where your boundaries were crossed or you were coerced or forced into any acts that you did not give consent to. You have the right to safe, sane, and consensual sex. If ever that isn't the case, I urge you to tell someone you trust and find ways to take care of yourself.

SAY IT OR SHOW IT?

Some of my clients feel overwhelmed by the idea that they have to communicate everything they want to a partner verbally. I often explain that there is a wide range of ways to communicate sexually. Not every sexual misfire needs to be talked about. In fact, nonverbal communication can be a valuable tool for getting things back on track. Using your body to signal what you like and don't like can be a great way to tell your partner something without stepping out of the moment too much. Here are some common nonverbal communication moves that can give your partner just the right amount of feedback.

Wrong Spot!

Not everyone will know your unique pleasure spots. It's important for arousal that you direct your partner to where on your body you get the most stimulation. You can guide them, with your hand over their hand, to move in ways that feel better for you than what they're doing.

Wrong Hole!

Sometimes there are innocent slipups and things can go places you'd rather they didn't. Use your hand to redirect the hand, penis, dildo, vibrator, etc. toward where you would prefer.

Finger Foul

Sometimes partners will use too many fingers or penetrate too deeply or too roughly for comfort or pleasure. Guide their hand out, grab the amount of fingers you want, and guide them back in at the pace and depth that feels good for you. Believe it or not, this can be incredibly sexy!

Too Deep, Not Deep Enough

When the depth of penetration is off, you can change positions to explore different depths and angles. In the early stages of sex, it may take some experimenting together to find which positions feel good for both of you.

USING YOUR WORDS

Now that you have a few pointers on how to communicate feedback with your body, I'll guide you through specific things you can say if you need to address things verbally.

Sometimes nonverbal communication minimizes the awkwardness of sexual mishaps or eliminates it altogether. But what happens when there's more than just fumbling and awkwardness? When there's an elephant in the room and that elephant's name is Bad Sex?

Talking about what's not working may feel like a real mood killer, which is why so many people choose not to do it. Most of the time, though, someone will need a little guidance, because it is rare to find partners who know exactly what you want. So how do you provide feedback in the heat of the moment? Below are a few common scenarios where feedback is necessary, and some ways to talk your way through it to something better.

When You Are in Pain

Sometimes a simple "ow" is all you need to initiate a pause in whatever you're doing so you can find a better position or tell the person that what they were doing or how they were doing it caused you pain. All bodies are different, so you're just giving the other person some parameters to work within for your body to feel its best during sex. Some folks, especially those with injuries or chronic pain, know which positions will exacerbate pain and which are better. You can share this beforehand or address it if it comes up during sex. Sex should be fun and pain-free (unless pain is part of how you experience pleasure), so if you get any response from your partner other than understanding and accommodation, you can cut that experience short.

When You Want More of Something

Sometimes partners will do something amazing but for a short period of time and then move on to something else. When this happens, it can feel hard to interrupt the flow of things to course correct back to something you like better. This may not be a huge problem, but it may impact how aroused you get and trickle down to whether you are having as much fun as possible. When someone does something great, let them know "I like it when you do that," and if they start moving on to something else, suggest they "stay there" and reiterate that what they're doing is working for you. Most people love being told they're doing something right, and you can't fully convey that with a moan or a grunt of pleasure.

When You Want Something Different

Sex is a cocreated experience, but it can sometimes feel like one person isn't fully participating. Maybe they are immersed in something that feels good to them but doesn't feel great to you. Maybe you've been putting in lots of effort only to feel like the other person is along for the ride. There are so many reasons why this disconnect can occur, from nerves and fatigue to downright selfishness. If you find yourself not liking the vibe or what the other person is doing, you can simply say, "This isn't working for me." If you have something else you'd like, suggest it! If you just want whatever's happening to stop, that's okay too.

When You Don't Like the Specific Way They Do Something

Sexual feedback takes many forms, but delivering feedback about how someone does something might be the hardest. For this type of feedback to be good, it has to be specific. Say you've agreed to some spanking, and the other person is a bit too eager for your taste and you're not enjoying their intensity. Having specific feedback can be really helpful. Things like "softer please," or "I like to be spanked just on my ass cheeks. Everywhere else is off-limits," can give the person direction to rein it in. This type of feedback can also be given for general touch or kissing. Letting someone know that you like more pressure, less tongue, lighter strokes, less teeth, or whatever the case may be could transform the entire experience. If you're met with resistance, you can explain that you think you would like the act better if it was tweaked a bit. If they are unwilling to try, this may point to a larger sexual mismatch.

When Your Boundaries Are Crossed

If you have a sexual boundary that you've shared with a partner, there is no reason that they should engage in activities that would cross that line. If they try, you can remind them that certain things are off-limits and that you have already discussed this. You can also say, "That's my boundary and we need to stop." Sometimes folks get carried away in the moment, but if the response to your feedback is anything but an apology and adherence to your boundary moving forward, that's an indicator that this person isn't someone with whom you can safely assert boundaries, and therefore is not a good sexual partner for you.

THERE'S A TIME AND A PLACE

Some people believe there are strict rules about when and how you should talk about sex. Some think you shouldn't critique someone you just met because if it doesn't work immediately, it's not a match. Others believe that you can talk about sex while having sex but specific feedback is off-limits—just stick to dirty talk and call it a day. And I've already mentioned that a lot of people don't believe in talking about sex ever. I personally have an early-and-often policy when it comes to talking about sex. The early stages of becoming sexual with someone are often fraught with nerves and carryover behaviors from previous partners (if they've had any) or a general lack of sexual confidence. There really is a lot to talk about!

Bringing sex into the conversation early can help in a couple ways. It sets a tone of openness and it can help build anticipation. When you are okay talking about your turn-ons and what you don't like with a partner, you give more space for figuring out whether you're sexually compatible. Some folks like to sext with potential dates to see if they are into the same things and like each other's vibe before having in-person sex. This may or may not be your thing. You may choose to give yourself a little while before bringing up sex, and that's fine too. When you do, you will be planting a seed for your potential partner to get excited about. Mentioning sex and your specific turn-ons is a mighty powerful aphrodisiac and can help bridge the gap between never having discussed anything related to sex and actually having it.

And when it comes to sexual feedback, setting a precedent that it's a natural part of the dating process will help you find your best matches. People who are unwilling to receive genuine feedback might not work for you long term. There may be things that you don't notice about a person until you become physical. And feedback can start as soon as your first kiss.

Take my client Kyle. She had a promising video date with someone she was really excited to meet in person. They agreed to meet out at a trivia night the following weekend, where things continued to go fairly well. One thing led to another, and they found themselves making out on the stoop in front of her apartment. Before the first kiss, Kyle was super attracted to her date, but as they made out something felt off between them. He was aggressive in ways that made her uncomfortable. At one point, she started to pull away and he responded by pulling her closer. She was excited, but also a little scared. He towered over her, and she began thinking about the many ways this could go south quickly. She was even second-guessing her decision to let him walk her all the way home. When he asked if he could come up to her apartment, she said she didn't think it was a good idea since she had an early morning meeting.

She went upstairs and wrote me an email recapping everything that had happened and, in the process, was able to pinpoint why the night had devolved into something that had left her feeling mildly traumatized. In retrospect, he had seemed more aloof on their in-person date, like he was there but way more self-conscious than he was on their video date. She chalked this up to nerves, but that's what made the aggressive make-out so shocking. It seemed counter to how he had been all night. I told her she didn't have to communicate with this person ever again if she didn't want to—or, if she felt it would help her process everything, she could offer him some feedback. She decided to text him a couple days after their date to let him know that she wasn't interested in going out with him again. He said he was disappointed to hear that and that he had had a really nice time with her. Mustering a lot of courage, she said that she had enjoyed herself too, up until he walked her home.

"Oh no! I'm so sorry. Did I move too fast?" he asked.

"I just felt really uncomfortable during our make-out. And when I tried to pull away, it felt like you got more aggressive," she said.

"I'm really sorry, Kyle. I definitely misread the situation. Thank you for telling me."

"You're welcome."

"I appreciate the feedback. I had actually been told that I'm too passive by a couple of people I dated. I guess I over-corrected. I'm still trying to figure all of this out. I'm so sorry I made you feel uncomfortable."

I'm always proud of my clients, but Kyle addressing this situation head-on was truly amazing. When we met for our next session, we talked through how she was feeling about how everything went. First of all, she was pleased that he responded positively. In dating, it is rare that you get to have thoughtful, honest exchanges like this. And second, it didn't change how Kyle felt about this guy. In the aftermath of the date and debriefing, she realized that there were other mismatches along the way that she hadn't been able to process in the moment. I told her that this often happens and that she now had more information for her next series of dates. She said that she would notice more closely if she felt like the other person wasn't tuning into her and responding to her energy. This would be something to add to her red flags list.

Not all feedback has to happen in the moment. Sometimes you might leave a situation feeling like it wasn't great, but it isn't until much later that you realize exactly why. It will be up to you if you feel like delivering this feedback. It isn't easy! Sometimes it's helpful for clearing the air and moving on. Other times it's what keeps the momentum going.

Like with my client Tala, who had to give sexual feedback to someone after the first time they had sex. Tala was able to turn things around with someone they had been dating for a while but had only recently become sexual with. They were taking things slowly after an emotionally tumultuous situationship had run its course. We started working together about two months after they met their new partner, and during our first session together they were contemplating breaking things off.

"The sex was bad. And I don't mean your everyday, garden-variety awkward sex because it's the first time. I mean it was bad in ways I can't really even describe. I don't think we can come back from this," they said.

I asked Tala to try to recall how everything went down, and they quipped, "Well, first of all, they didn't go down!"

"Ahhhh. And was there anything else missing? How was what you ended up doing bad?" I asked.

They told me that their partner was rougher than they liked. Not rough as in dominant, actually rough—heavy-handed, rushed, and generally not in tune with how to touch them. When I asked if they'd had a conversation about what had happened with their partner, Tala paused and said, "I'm actually really good at feedback usually, but this was so off I didn't know where to start so I just bounced."

Tala thought they had done a good job of communicating what they liked and disliked and the fact that they needed a lot of buildup to any type of penetration. They said that these things had come up naturally when the two of them had discussed previous partners. Since they were recently single, Tala had really fresh information to share with their partner. "Were they just not listening to me?" they asked.

I told them that even though they were transparent about what they liked, it sometimes takes a few times to get on the same page about what those desires actually mean during sex. Perhaps there was a miscommunication, or in the heat of the moment their partner totally forgot any guidance that had been shared beforehand. Because Tala had started to develop feelings for this person, they found it hard to stop in the middle of sex to talk about what was going wrong. I encouraged them to do just that, in the interest of finding out if some real-time feedback could help.

On their next date, Tala opened up a little bit about how they really felt about that first sex attempt. Initially, this was met with some resistance. "But you didn't say anything. I thought we both had fun." Tala shared that they had been at a loss for words in the moment and then reiterated the things they needed for arousal, which included oral sex, softer touch, and going a lot slower than they had before. Tala's partner responded with, "Okay, I guess I remember that you like things slow. I kinda just got swept up in the moment."

They both agreed to stay open to in-the-moment feedback and, after a few sessions in which Tala reminded their partner to slow down, the two of them began to find their rhythm. The addition of oral sex to the mix didn't hurt either. Tala guided their partner to areas of their body that were the most arousing for them, and they were able to relax and enjoy everything else from that point on.

"I know that not everyone is going to know how I like sex. I had just never encountered this type of misalignment before. It was a shock to recognize that even though I felt like I was setting myself up for success, I could still have to work with someone to really get what I need from the experience. But it felt good! We're getting better together. They even gave *me* some feedback the other day, and I had to be like, 'Okay, tell me how I can make this better for you,'" Tala said.

Tala's a great example of normalizing talking about sex as part of the dating process. Sometimes that's enough, and sometimes you'll need in-the-moment communication and even follow-up conversations. If bringing sex into everyday conversation feels like a bit much, you can start by expanding how much you talk about sex around the act itself. You can start to communicate what you want before, during, and after sex in straightforward and simple ways. Here are a few suggestions for how to structure those conversations during each time frame.

Before Sex

- Describe likes and dislikes. There's nothing wrong with telling someone your favorite position or things you'd like to avoid.

- Have a consent conversation. What activities are both of you into? Are there any STIs that need to be disclosed prior to consenting to certain acts?

During Sex

- Use your body. Remember those nonverbal cues that can help move things along. Don't be afraid to guide your partner toward what you like.

- Highlight what's working. Use positive reinforcement for things you enjoy and give constructive feedback about things you don't.

After Sex

- Check in. See how they're feeling and let them know how you're feeling after sex.

- Have a debrief conversation. What did each of you like? Are there things that you'd tweak in hindsight?

EXERCISE: YOUR IDEAL
SEXUAL EXPERIENCE

Based on what you know about yourself from masturbation and your sexual values, what would make sex truly mind-blowing for you? What are the conditions that would make you feel comfortable, confident, and super sexy? Are there any themes or words that pop up frequently that you can use to help describe what you want?

Now take a moment to consider when you can share this information with a partner. Can you incorporate your wants and needs into conversations about past relationships? Can you advocate for your pleasure in the moment by delivering nonverbal or verbal sexual feedback? Pick one way you can work on being a better sexual communicator.

Sexual communication, particularly feedback, is one way we can deepen our connection to others. When we have a need that we feel we can express and have met by someone else, it's exhilarating. But most of us have little experience with this type of communication, and it can be daunting to have to tell another person exactly what you want and how.

Partners who are invested in a mutually pleasurable experience will be open to learning more about how your body works and what it needs to feel its best in sexual situations. You can build up your knowledge of yourself so that when there is a misalignment or you have to deliver feedback, you have the words to describe what you need, which makes the process a little easier. Sexual communication is a skill we all have to develop, so practice makes it easier over time.

11

Exiting the Apps Gracefully

Leave the party while you're still having fun.
—PARTY ADAGE

Hopefully you have some newfound clarity about what you can say to partners to make the most of all of your sexual experiences from here on out. Maybe you were even able to deliver some much needed sexual feedback and it resulted in a better sexual experience for all parties involved. And maybe, because of your bravery in speaking up for yourself and your needs, you're more hopeful about dating as a whole.

You may have even decided by this point to focus on one or a few connections you've made to see how they'll develop. This is an interesting place to arrive. It's often the destination for a lot of my clients—a place where they can settle into getting to know folks better by spending more time together, all while revealing more about themselves in the process. But this stage of dating isn't without its complexities. There are lots of emotions that get stirred up by the prospect of investing more in other people sexually and/or romantically, and that can lead to questions like: How much is too much time to give to someone? How many people should I date at once? And when exactly should I leave the apps?

In dating, there's a perception that things are the most complicated and draining when they're going horribly wrong, but sometimes things are even more complicated when they're going right. Earlier, we covered how using dating apps can contribute to burnout and how to recognize when it's time to take a break. Unfortunately, burnout is a common and maddening part of the dating process. It can be disillusioning if you invest time and energy into dating and it doesn't deliver what you want in return. That's when it's easy to think that the smart move is to disengage from dating altogether and give yourself a break. But sometimes it's a good idea to end your relationship with the apps on a high note—when you're actually feeling like the process *is* working.

Understanding how dating negatively or positively affects your energy and choices is an important part of making the most of the experience. When you're enjoying yourself, it can be difficult to recognize when to give yourself a break to soak up all of that positive energy and let things move at their own pace. It can also be hard to believe that you're actually getting what you wanted. In Chapter 8, we went over how Bigger Better Deal Syndrome can keep you in a dating loop unnecessarily. BBDS tends to pop up when you have one or more exciting prospects to pursue, but you just aren't convinced that you're on the right track. Modern dating is full of mental traps like this that we occasionally fall into. Another common trap is believing that to get *exactly* what you want, you just have to keep on dating. With that mindset, it's easy to get caught up in what could be and lose sight of what is. In other words, it's hard to know if you're having fun if you're preoccupied by the fun you might have with people you haven't met yet.

In this chapter, we'll explore the benefits of moving on once you've found yourself somehow, miraculously, having a good time. Sometimes concentrating on the connections you've made just makes more sense than seeking out new ones, and that's when it's time to say goodbye to the apps. Their siren song can be so strong though! So we'll cover how to determine the right time to leave, whether to tell the people you're dating that you're off the apps, and how you can do that confidently without feeling like you're missing out. We'll even explore some very good reasons why you might find yourself hesitant to leave the apps and why staying put could be best for you.

LIMIT YOUR DISTRACTIONS

New connections require your attention. One benefit of leaving the apps once you've met people you are excited about is that you limit the distractions that may keep you from fully learning about these people and assessing whether you meet each other's needs. Stepping back from the apps at this point could keep you from experiencing dating burnout. Think about all of the attention that apps require of you and how much time is spent just swiping and hoping for matches. It doesn't feel particularly productive to be giving your time away to the apps when you have people you want to spend time with in person.

Most dating apps use gamification strategies—they maximize your engagement with them by making you feel like you could "win" dating by getting matches, which is not usually the goal for most people. Most folks are looking to share experiences by meeting in person, but the apps weren't designed to encourage you to find what you're looking for then leave. This is true for pretty much all dating apps and sites, despite any claims that they were made to be deleted.

You would think that limiting distractions would be enough incentive to disengage from the apps, but it's usually not. For many, the activity of dating is closely connected to the game of chance that dating apps ensnare them in, and it's hard to know when to stop swiping and let in-person relationships begin.

Take my client Sahara. She and I started working together when she was ready to prioritize dating but wasn't quite sure how to start. As a single mom, she had given so much of her time and attention to her career and family over the last decade that online dating felt foreign, intimidating, and demoralizing. She worked hard on her profile and put her truth of being ready to find a loving long-term partner out there. She ended up really hitting it off with a father of two who was going through a divorce. He was a breath of fresh air compared to a lot of the elusive men she had dated in the past. The more time they spent together, the more she realized how much she liked him. He not only was consistent and treated her as an equal, which were really strong values for her, but he was a great match sexually and understood her time constraints as a working mom. Sahara was not prepared for this. Shouldn't it have taken longer? Could she really be heading toward the relationship she wanted after only a few months of searching?

In one of our sessions, she mentioned that she thought that she and her partner were on the verge of defining the relationship. I asked her how she felt about that, and she shared that she was excited and scared. She knew that her guy wasn't dating anyone else because he told her so after a few dates.

"Does that mean that I shouldn't be dating anyone else either?" she asked.

"Not necessarily," I began. "It really depends on how you're feeling and what you want from the situation."

It was then that she confessed, "I want this man to be my boyfriend. I hate that word, but you know what I mean. I want to be his focus and I want him to be my focus."

"That's great! Sounds like you're ready to deactivate your apps."

There was a long pause. Then she said, "Oh. I guess I should, right?"

I reminded Sahara about how she'd felt when we first started working together, how she had lamented having to use apps to find a partner. Now she was finding it hard to let go and be fully present for the person who might be that partner, even though the apps hadn't produced any other matches she was excited about.

By leaving the apps and limiting her distractions, Sahara found that she could ease her way into the role of "girlfriend"—a role she hadn't had since college. She became more focused on how the relationship was growing between them and even let herself get excited about milestones like meeting each other's friends, kids, and family. The two were starting to consider trips away together, which was very new and something she hadn't let herself think about as a possibility before. Though all of this was what Sahara had wanted when we started working together, she had become accustomed to having the apps there in the event that things didn't work out. It wasn't totally obvious to her to close them down until I brought the idea to her attention.

If you have been in a similar situation—where you felt good about what you had but scared about what comes next—I want to acknowledge how common it is. Too often, folks forget that the apps are just tools to help them find the kinds of connections they're looking for. So let this be a reminder: you don't have to maintain an ongoing relationship with dating apps once you have found something that works for you, whether that's a few great sexual partners, an activity buddy, fun dates, or a potential long-term relationship. Disengaging from the apps is the next step in making the shift from seeking to enjoying what you've got!

Also, your time is a limited resource, so if you're finding that you don't have enough time to give to the person, or people, you're interested in pursuing, it's a good move to exit the apps. Sometimes this will sneak up on you. Things will be going smoothly until a couple extra dates, a big work deadline, and a family obligation all hit around the same time. It's not always sustainable to keep adding new partners to the mix, because even though those initial connections can be fun, they are also a lot to manage emotionally. From first-date nerves, to figuring out how you feel about a person, to deciding how and where they might fit into your life, each step involves a bit of your time and consideration.

Even the most seasoned daters have their limits! So think about yours.

NARROW IT DOWN

Eventually the pool of options you started with will get smaller and smaller as you learn and refine what you're looking for. This narrowing down is what all that swiping and matching and going on dates is for. So why is it so scary to put the phone down and ride things out? First of all, it feels really vulnerable to act in ways that show you like someone. Shutting down the apps is one way you can signify to yourself and other people that you aren't interested in anything new right now. For a lot of folks, admitting that they're into someone (even to themself) is really hard. Second, it can be anxiety inducing to think that by quitting the apps you may be missing out on "better" people. Vulnerability plus anxiety equals a difficult headspace to be in, and some folks would rather keep the apps running in the background than face these unpleasant feelings.

This was definitely the case with my client Annie, who was overwhelmed by the idea that she could be happy enough with the partners she had. Her recently opened marriage gave her new freedoms she had never experienced before. She was actually one of my clients who loved dating for dating's sake, but she struggled with narrowing down how many relationships she could realistically handle at one time. She was, after all, only one person—and a busy one at that. Her excitement for and openness to new people and experiences made it hard for her to pause and evaluate how each relationship was developing on its own. She also loved just messaging back and forth with people, but that was starting to feel more like a chore.

Even with months of experiences under her belt and multiple burgeoning relationships, Annie was hesitant to give up the chase. The problem arose when one of her partners let her know that they had exited the apps and wanted to see where her head was at about deepening their relationship and spending more time together. They knew that Annie had other partners and that she was a self-proclaimed flirt, but they wondered if they could get what they needed from her when she was still focused on filling up her schedule with first dates. This was when Annie had her day of reckoning with the apps.

"I think I need to quit the apps for a while, and it's kinda stressing me out," she began one session.

"Oh? What changed?" I asked.

She told me about the heart-to-heart she'd had with her partner and how it had helped her realize how fortunate she was to have not only a loving wife but several new partners with whom she was learning so much. She said, "I guess when I started dating I wasn't expecting to find what I was looking for, if that makes sense. I also just love meeting new people, which I realize now could go on forever unless I put some parameters around it. It's hard to come to terms with the fact that I have this amazing community already and that it's through them—not the apps—that I'm enjoying myself the most. Before my partner said something, I was still thinking of everything as fleeting. It didn't matter if I was all over the place because I thought everyone else I was seeing was too.

But my goal was to find people to date, not continuously flirt with no expectations."

"I think it's a good idea to give yourself some time and space to develop what you have in the interest of not losing it. Maybe down the line you'll have more space to explore beyond these relationships again."

Annie agreed and broke out her phone. "Let me just rip the Band-Aid off right now." While she deleted her apps, she said it was kind of sad to be moving on but also really freeing to know that she had a lot to look forward to. I reminded her that, just as her expectations had changed over the months she was dating, they could also change as she took time away from the apps to learn more about herself and her relationships. A break could give her the necessary space to prioritize and see what relationships will and won't work for her long term.

EXERCISE: CHECKING IN ON YOUR PROGRESS

What's your best-case scenario when it comes to dating? Is it that you have a primary partner and a couple others who you see occasionally? Is it that you find one person with whom you share a strong enough connection that a long-term relationship emerges? Is it to have a steady stream of dates, hookups, and noncommittal connections? Think back to those three-, six-, and twelve-month goals you created for yourself. Has anything changed significantly? Are you getting closer to what you wanted? Take a moment to check in with yourself and note how dating has been treating you so far.

What has surprised you most about dating this time around? Who has surprised you? What's your biggest win? Are you living your best-case scenario, given what you wanted and the experiences you've had?

Noticing how far you've progressed is helpful when deciding if it's time to quit the apps. It's easy to lose sight of what you wanted when you started dating, especially if you've been staying open throughout the process, so I recommend doing this kind of check-in every month or so to chart your progress.

DIGISEXUALITY AND OTHER REASONS TO STAY CONNECTED TO THE APPS

Not everyone who dates is looking for exclusively in-person experiences. For some folks, online dating and relationships that are mediated by some form of technology are the most fulfilling. They may prefer messaging through the apps, texting, and video chat over in-person dates and feel the most at home sexually if there's a piece of technology involved. Whether it's through sexting, camming, watching porn online, or using sex dolls, AI, or other tech during sex and masturbation, digisexuals enjoy the fact that sex can be technologically savvy.

If this feels like you, then you may identify as digisexual.* You might also find it hard to disengage from app-based

---

* Neil McArthur and Markie L. C. Twist, "The Rise of Digisexuality: Therapeutic Challenges and Possibilities," *Sexual and Relationship Therapy* 32, no. 3–4 (February 2017): 334–344, https://doi.org/10.108 0/14681994.2017.1397950.

dating because of this. And that's fine. Feel free to add this to your profile if you find it helpful or let people know what you're looking for when you match with them. It might help you to develop more satisfying relationships with people who also want tech-mediated experiences.

Digisexuality is one reason to remain on the apps. Another is app-based dating's ability to provide community. This can happen for singles or folks in relationships. For instance, I have encountered couples for whom exiting the apps never happens. They are content to continue to meet people online, possibly moving those interactions to in-person meetings. Some relationships include space for exploring and building a wider community through app-based connections. Take John and Jason, who met on a popular gay dating app and never felt the need to leave, even after they became an official couple. Though not in a completely open relationship, they both derived joy from meeting other gay men in their city and strengthening their community ties there. Sometimes there was flirting, sometimes not. They would often show each other the guys they were connecting with and weigh in on each other's matches. Using apps in this way can work for all types of relationships, but it appeals predominantly to those who are monogamish, polyamorous, kinky, or just in search of other folks with whom they share an identity.

If you like to use apps in this way, that's something you can negotiate with a partner. Lots of apps have an option for "friends only" or some variation that indicates your intentions. You can also choose to use social media or other networking apps to foster these types of connections. The fact that some folks remain on dating sites in search of community well after they have found romantic partnership points to a general trend of finding any and all human connections through technology. So whether digisexuality feels right to you or you just want to continue to find other people with whom you have things in common, dating apps could be a way that you get your connection needs met.

GETTING ON THE SAME PAGE

When it comes to focusing on the people you're already seeing, sometimes it will be obvious when you're on the same page as them and sometimes it won't be as clear. For some of my clients, it takes a few hard but clarifying conversations to help them see that they're actually quite happy to step back from the apps. For other clients, no conversation is required. They met people they liked, disengaged from swiping, and just enjoyed their relationships from there.

But there are times when not everyone wants the same things, or at least not at the exact same time. You might find yourself ready to go all-in on a relationship—whether you've found your perfect sexual match, someone with whom you see long-term potential, or someone you're just intrigued to learn more about—and they may want to continue dating around. Or it may be you who turns down the invitation to commit more time to someone because you're not ready or you have other needs that aren't being met by the people you're seeing. This happens a lot, so it's good to remember that each person is coming to the experience with not only their own set of values and things that they're looking for but also a history of past relationships, doubts, and fears that could impact how much they can give to the people they're dating. These factors often determine whether people feel ready to leave the apps.

The classic, but very limiting, way we view this type of scenario is that if one person wants more exclusivity and the other person isn't ready, then it's a bad match. The idea is that if you stick around while someone figures out how they feel about you, then you're settling. But the reality is usually more complex than that. It would be great to always feel in sync with the people who give us the most pleasure—to progress in each relationship at the same pace and never question the bonds that form—but that's impossible even in the steadiest relationships.

We ask a lot of ourselves and others when we insist on being "ready" when great people come around, and this type of pressure is what causes us to either be overlooked or overlook others as potential matches. The reality is that there are a lot of things that could intervene in our ability to progress our relationships, like inexperience, nursing a recent heartbreak, figuring out your sexuality, or struggling with a mental or physical health issue. All of these could put limits on how much a person can give to someone else. You may have gone through periods of dating when something like this was a factor in whether or not you pursued a relationship, so it's good to keep an open mind if you encounter others who aren't yet "ready" to commit more to you.

Does this mean you should wait around forever for someone who doesn't want as much from the relationship as you do? Absolutely not. It means that if a person isn't ready to move things forward on your timeline, it's good to get a better understanding of why this is the case and decide if that's a factor you can work with. You can't make someone fit exactly into your timeline, but you can control your own actions. If you feel a connection is worth focusing on, you can decide to drop the apps without holding the other person to the same standard. The main thing is to be confident in your own decision to leave the apps. You can't make that decision for others, but you can begin to examine the relationship based on whether they are ready to leave the apps with you.

This is what my client Hayden did after months of dating a few people at a time. As someone who hadn't dated around or had much sex in her twenties, she wanted to feel more experienced before hitting her thirties. She did not expect to be in a position to turn people down who wanted relationships, but that's exactly what she did throughout her work with me. She kept her eye on her goals of figuring out what she liked sexually and trying to find partners with whom she clicked, no strings attached. For the most part, she was happy with the experiences she had, and she felt like she had learned a lot even in the times that weren't so fun. But in one session, she told me that she felt she was falling for one of the guys she had been dating.

"I'm off the apps as of today," she explained. "This feels really different, in a good way, and I want to see where it goes."

She told me that the object of her affection was actually a coworker who had recently broken up with his partner of several years. They had always been friendly, chatting together during after-hours office functions, and when he became single they started hooking up.

"He's on another team and our work doesn't really overlap. Beyond work we have a lot in common! We come from very similar immigrant, Midwestern backgrounds, and he's just super easy to open up to. That's something that felt really different from my other hookups." She said that she quietly exited the apps and wasn't intending to tell her partner, partially because she wasn't ready to but primarily because she knew he was still going through the fallout of his breakup. She didn't want to put any undue pressure on him and she understood that he was probably making good use of being single again.

As time went on, Hayden continued to enjoy their friends-with-benefits situation. They had a good thing going that she didn't put too many expectations on, given what she knew her guy was capable of. This worked for a few months before she realized she was ready for something deeper. When she shared her feelings, he told her that he still wasn't in a place to start a relationship. Though it was difficult to talk through, his response wasn't completely unexpected. Once she got confirmation that they weren't on the same page emotionally, she decided to move on from that relationship. By giving herself some time to develop feelings, Hayden had gotten a better sense of what she now wanted and was actually better prepared to reenter dating. When she started up the apps again, her focus was on finding a long-term relationship with someone she could develop a friendship with and who could relate to her background and upbringing.

HOW TO HANDLE AN
EXPECTATION MISMATCH

It's okay if you end up connecting with people here and there who aren't on the same page as you when it comes to dating expectations. It doesn't mean you won't learn, grow, or even enjoy yourself as things progress with someone who wants different things than you. But it's important to keep tabs on how you feel along the way. Are you getting what you need from the experience? Are you open to seeing how things evolve, or are you ready for more certainty?

There will likely be a time when someone you're seeing shares that they've left the apps, or maybe you notice this on your own because your match disappears and their profile is gone. It can feel like a lot of pressure to know that someone has left the apps when you're content to stay on. Or, on the flip side, you could jump to the conclusion that they want to be exclusive because they've left the apps when that couldn't be further from the truth.

The best way to handle a mismatch is to talk about it. Letting things progress when you know you're not on the same page as your partner can be a real bummer later. It's best to talk through what each of you is thinking so you can both have clarity. I've compiled a list of reasons why someone may be feeling the itch to ditch before you so you can talk through what's going on and let them know how you're feeling as well.

Below are some common reasons people quit the apps after meeting you:

- They really like you. Leaving the apps has become an official sign of interest in modern dating. Does it mean you have to do the same? Only if you're ready.

- Dating sucks. Sometimes people want to make things official and leave the apps because they just hate dating. This can contribute to hasty decision-making or pressure on the other person to make a decision before they're ready to. If you feel pressure to move faster than you're comfortable with, let the other person know that you aren't ready to leave the apps just yet.

- They have dating anxiety. People who get overwhelmed easily by dating may opt out sooner than those who don't totally hate the process. It doesn't necessarily mean that they want to go all in; they may just want to limit their distractions, and one person at a time is really all they can handle.

ARE YOU READY TO SAY GOODBYE?

Think about how you feel when you use the apps versus when you are with the people you're dating. Which causes more stress and anxiety? Why?

If you've made a few good connections, how would it feel to focus on those for a while? And if someone seems ready to go deeper with you, is that something you want right now? If not, what would feel better?

When you're having a good time dating, it can be hard to recognize when you've reached one of the goals you were striving for when you started the process. Whether you're casually seeing multiple people or you've decided that prioritizing the connection you've made with one person is how you'd like to spend your time, exiting the apps might be right for you. The benefits of stepping away from the apps once you've found something that feels good include limiting your distractions so you can feel more present and available and narrowing down your choices as your relationship(s) unfold over time. When you decide to leave the apps, be sure it's because you want to, and let the folks you're seeing make that decision in their own time as well.

12

The Magical Art of Breaking Up

The way they leave tells you everything.

—RUPI KAUR

Although it's fun to focus on all of the new beginnings of dating, we rarely discuss the many difficult endings that can occur and what to do about them. Try as you might to achieve all of your dating goals and solidify connections with amazing people, unless you are incredibly lucky, you will experience at least one, if not many, breakups along the way. These can range from cordial conversations where you mutually agree to part ways to painful separations from people you've become emotionally attached to. And whether you are the instigator of a breakup or on the receiving end, the general consensus is that it's the shittiest part of dating. There's really no sugarcoating it.

In fact, fear of breakups is a really common reason people opt out of dating. Breaking up is hard! And some folks have a difficult time getting back into dating once they've felt the sting of heartbreak. While there's no way to completely avoid this, I hope it helps to know that pretty much everyone goes through it and most folks come out of breakups with a better understanding of who they are as a partner and what they want from relationships in the future. Think of it this way: a breakup is like a burn, and when you heal from it, you're a little tougher and wiser.

Of course, there are run-of-the-mill breakups that most people bounce back from, and there are life-changing breakups after being mistreated by a partner. Leaving an abusive, coercive, or toxic relationship can be a long and emotional process in and of itself. And healing from these types of relationships often requires some outside support in the form of counseling, therapy, or recovery groups. If you find yourself questioning whether you're in an unhealthy relationship, I urge you to talk to someone, even just a close friend, about it. Reaching out might be the first step in exiting a toxic situation and beginning the healing process. If you're feeling stuck while dating because of a past bad relationship, I hope you'll seek some support as well. Dating can stir up lots of emotions, and it could really make a difference for you to have someone you can talk to along the way.

Generally speaking, we could all do a better job at breakups, but most of us don't have a good model for this. Instead, we witnessed the painful and sometimes vindictive process of divorce in our families or watched as friends went through nasty breakups, never to speak their ex's name again. We may have even taken part in some foul breakup behavior ourselves. And honestly, why wouldn't we? Without envisioning what breakups could be or seeing them as opportunities to be kind and grow, it's hard to navigate them in the moments when tensions and emotions are so high. Of course there are those for whom breaking up wasn't the end of the relationship. We see this in folks who were able to build lifelong friendships with each other after parting ways as partners. Not every breakup is made for this, but I believe that there's plenty of space between hating each other's guts and friends forever; in that space we can all do our part to leave things a little better.

In this chapter, we'll focus on ways to navigate breakups more smoothly. You'll learn the signs that it might be time to exit your relationship and how to communicate how you're feeling. I'll also cover how to create a breakup plan for yourself so you can feel more confident when the time comes to move on.

Are you ready to get into the not-so-fun stuff? With some guidance, I have no doubt that you'll be better prepared when endings eventually happen and more able to accept breakups as a growth opportunity for everyone involved.

HOW TO KNOW WHEN IT'S OVER

Many of my clients find it difficult to call a relationship quits, even when they have a sinking feeling that things have run their course. As previously mentioned, breakups suck regardless of who initiates them, so it doesn't surprise me when folks try to avoid a potentially painful situation for as long as possible. It's also common for it to take a bit of time to sort through everything that pre-breakup thoughts stir up. Do you really want to break up, or are you terrified of trusting another person? Is the other person acting distant because they want to leave you, or are they bad at communicating when their life gets really stressful? Are you not sexually attracted to them anymore, or is this something you can both work on together? The list of possible explanations for that sinking feeling is incredibly long. So how do you know if what you're feeling is actually a good reason to break up with someone?

It will probably come as no surprise to you when I say that talking about what you're feeling is a good way to figure all of this out. Sometimes talking to a friend, especially if that friend has perspective on your relationship history, can help you sort things out. And sometimes you have to talk through what you're thinking with your partner directly, which can feel like a lot, especially if you're not sure if you want to break up yet. But if you can't talk openly about how you see the relationship going, that might be the very sign that you need to break up!

My client Kalise ran into this issue after dating someone for about six months. She really wanted things to work out between them, but she was starting to feel a bit apprehensive. In the beginning of their relationship, things moved so quickly and smoothly that she found herself settling into a rhythm with her partner sooner than she had in previous relationships. She was also able to open up and express her feelings for him in ways she hadn't before. It felt new and exciting to connect with someone who was very clear about wanting the same things as she did: to be married, start a family, and be bicoastal. With most of her family on the other side of the country, it was important for her to feel that she could split her time, and she dreamed of having a partner who was open to this possible future too.

Because of the pandemic, things between them had progressed quickly and they were already discussing moving in together. Those conversations were tough because she could sense his discomfort with talking about money—something that was pretty important when it came to deciding where they could both afford to rent. At that point, Kalise started to reflect more deeply on other areas of their relationship that were strained. Their sex life, for instance, was something she wanted to work on, but he retreated from any suggestion that they should address this together. She was noticing a pattern. It actually only felt easy to open up to her partner when she kept conversations to things he was willing to discuss. This, she told me in one session, was not going to work for her long term. "If we can't talk about the hard stuff now, how is that going to play out in the future if we start a family? Are things just going to be on his terms all the time? That's not an equal partnership. I get it, this stuff is hard and I don't like talking about it either, but we have to work on our communication or I don't think this is the relationship for me," she said.

Kalise was caught in a moment when she could either commit further to her relationship or leave it altogether. It was make-or-break time. She decided to be open about her concerns with her partner, and while he could admit that communication wasn't his strength, he still believed that the relationship was working just fine. That's when Kalise suggested that they consider couples therapy to help them both address some of the more challenging topics he tended to avoid. Unfortunately, her partner rejected that idea and told her that if they needed to work on things this early in the relationship, it probably didn't bode well for their future. Both of them were coming to a similar conclusion about where things were heading, but for very different reasons.

Sometimes breakups will unfold like this. As one person notices and points out something that isn't quite working for them, the other person has the chance to address these concerns. As much as they cared for each other, Kalise and her partner were at an impasse. She needed him to be more proactive in learning better communication skills, and he was hesitant to commit more to a relationship that he thought was built on a mismatch. But there are times when it's harder to see where the disconnect is. In fact, most of the time, breakups begin with a vague feeling.

There are a few common signs that may indicate your relationship is in question and might be headed toward a breakup. These signs can be internal feelings or doubts about the relationship or a pattern of behaviors and actions that you or your partner show over time. Taken on their own, they might just be natural snags as you get to know each other, but combined and persistent feelings and actions like the ones below are good indicators that there's something wrong. I've listed some signs that at the very least a conversation is needed, and at the absolute worst may mean a breakup is near.

Internal Feelings

- Feeling unsure about how much you like this person
- Not feeling as attracted to them as you used to be
- Feeling uncomfortable or unlike yourself when you're together

- Feeling like you don't have much in common
- Not seeing a future with this person or feeling too much pressure to plan when you're not ready

Behaviors

- Not being as responsive to communications as in the past
- Pulling back on signs of affection like hugs, kisses, and compliments
- Shutting down when talks about the future come up or avoiding these conversations altogether
- Not checking in with or thinking about the other person that much
- Backing out of dates last minute with no clear reason

If you find yourself having a lot of the feelings on the first list, you could actually be doing things on the second list without being consciously aware of it. And if you notice your partner is doing a lot of the things on the bottom list, they may be thinking about the things on the top list.

It's helpful to recognize these signals, not because they always mean the end of the relationship, but because acknowledging behaviors and feelings will help you be more intentional about how you communicate what's going on with your partner. Without a clear view of what you're feeling, or what behaviors are causing you concern, it's very hard to start a conversation.

EXERCISE: WHAT'S MISSING FROM
YOUR CONNECTION?

Making the decision to end a relationship—no matter how long you've known someone and how close you are—is never easy. It's good to give yourself some time to process what it is that you're missing. Is it passion, intimacy, shared interests, sexual values, or communication? Get clear about what you're not getting and why it's important. Are these concerns something that you believe you can work on? Why or why not?

If your connection is strong now, you can revisit this exercise later if things start to feel unsteady.

TIPS FOR COMMUNICATING
YOUR RELATIONSHIP NEEDS

If you notice feelings popping up that give you pause about the relationship, it could be really helpful to share them, if for no other reason than to let the other person in on how you're doing. One of the benefits of being in a partnership is that you have someone who cares about you and what you're feeling. Sometimes our feelings are indicative of an insecurity we feel in the relationship, and sometimes they point to a larger issue. For instance, recognizing that someone isn't responding to your texts as quickly as they used to can stir up a lot of emotions. In your anxiety, you might jump to conclusions and throw out accusations, while the other person is unaware that their behavior is having a negative effect. Or they might be dealing with something else that they have been hesitant to bring up with you, so they've been slower to engage with you. If you feel like something is off, there's a way you can communicate that without having the situation go off the rails and result in the person totally missing the point that their behavior is having a negative effect on your relationship.

For these conversations, it's helpful to use the Situation-Behavior-Impact (SBI) feedback model.* This is often used in leadership communication, but is a great tool for pretty much any tough conversation. The situation includes specifics about what you've observed in the relationship and when. For example, a change in mood or behaviors that make you nervous or uncomfortable and how long it has been this way. Follow this with a summary of the behavior that you've noticed in your partner. Try to be as specific as possible when describing these behaviors, listing any patterns that have emerged that might be helpful for them to know. Then state the impact that this behavior has had on you or the health of the relationship.

Below I've listed some ways for bringing your observations to light using the SBI framework, which can help you structure hard conversations without getting too overwhelmed. Keep in mind that these conversations could result in the other person confirming that what you're feeling is a sign that the relationship is on its last legs, or they might just learn more about how you interpret their behavior and how

---

* Leading Effectively Staff, "How to Use Situation-Behavior-Impact (SBI) to Explore Intent vs. Impact," Center for Creative Leadership, November 18, 2020, www.ccl.org/articles/leading-effectively-articles /closing-the-gap-between-intent-vs-impact-sbii.

the things they have done affect you. Try to stay open to all possible outcomes.

> **Situation:** This past month it feels like we haven't been connecting.
> **Behavior:** I've noticed that you don't text back like you used to, sometimes ignoring questions I ask you.
> **Impact:** I'm feeling unsure about where I stand with you.

> **Situation:** Over the last few weeks we've only seen each other a couple times.
> **Behavior:** You've canceled plans last minute three times.
> **Impact:** It feels like something's wrong and you're avoiding me.

But what if it's you who is pulling away or starting to doubt the relationship? Here are a couple examples of what to say to share your feelings using the SBI framework. It's a good idea to address these concerns once you really feel them becoming an issue in your relationship. For instance, if your doubts are causing you to put off or cancel plans with your partner, it's best to share how you've been feeling and point out how this has been impacting your own behavior.

> **Situation:** I haven't felt like myself these past couple weeks.
> **Behavior:** I've been really anxious on our last few dates and haven't been able to enjoy myself.
> **Impact:** I'm not sure that this is the right relationship for me.

Situation: These past few days, I've been thinking about our relationship.

Behavior: The huge fight we had last week made me realize how different we both are and how we need different things.

Impact: I think we need to break up.

Using the SBI framework can help you start a hard conversation when it feels impossible to do so. It can also help you sort out how you're feeling and be clear about how you see what's happening in the relationship. Additionally, SBI is great to use if you start feeling that urge to ghost. Rather than pull a disappearing act, take some time to gather your thoughts and write out your feelings.

If you're in the midst of a relationship make-or-break moment, take a few minutes to consider how you might start a conversation with your partner about what's going on. Have you noticed situations, behaviors, and impacts that have concerned you? If you're not there yet, remember that the SBI model is here for you when you need it.

*

How to Address When You Want to Date Other People in Addition to Your Current Partner

Sometimes breaking up isn't the intended outcome of pointing out what's not working in the relationship. You may be curious about what it would be like to have an open relationship or are practicing nonmonogamy but have been focusing on only one relationship for a time. In these cases, you have to communicate to your partner that, in addition to being with them, you would like to explore connections with other people. Depending on your partner and their needs, this can feel like a breakup or, in cases where being in an open relationship isn't on the table, it can become a breakup conversation.

Part of determining whether your relationship can survive opening up is having a dialogue about what each of you wants from the relationship you already have. Some of my clients find themselves at a crossroads and both parties can clearly see the benefit of maintaining their connection while pursuing other people. It energizes them individually to have other partners and they find that nonmonogamy even deepens their relationship to each other. Other clients have explored being open and find that they both actually want to leave the relationship and either be single again or date around and learn more about themselves. The conversation about being open was a way for them to start talking more about their needs. In the end, they learned that they needed very different things.

For these conversations to go as smoothly as possible, you need to be very clear about what you want from dating other people in addition to your current partner. Not sure? Take a few minutes to envision what your ideal scenario would look like. Do you both date other people? Are other relationships only casual or would you like several long-term relationships developing at the same time? If casual is the goal, how will you go about this safely so that your partner feels comfortable? Are there any people who are off-limits, like friends, exes, coworkers, etc.? There are many ways to be nonmonogamous, so if you haven't given this much thought, I recommend reading up on the various ways that open relationships can be structured so you can communicate your needs to your partner effectively.

*

My client Carlo used the SBI framework to talk about a misalignment between him and his partner after a couple months of dating. It was becoming clear to him that the two of them viewed sex very differently. Carlo and I began working together because he was tired of hooking up and wanted something more consistent, long-term, and sexually satisfying. He was instantly drawn to his new partner because, on top of being incredibly attracted to one another, they both shared a desire to settle down and start a family. Carlo was excited by the fact that they were both ready to leave the apps and focus on building a deeper relationship. He was intrigued by how attentive and affectionate his partner was, and he loved how romantic their dates felt. There was just one thing that gave him pause.

"Myisha, it's been two months and we haven't had sex," Carlo told me. "Am I the worst if I say this is totally not okay?"

I explained that he might be taken aback by someone who wants to focus on creating an emotional connection first. His past experiences started out very physical, so this was all new territory. He agreed that this felt different, and it had given him hope that he could find a partner who was more serious about him and his needs.

"But what if he's really bad at sex? What if we have zero compatibility in bed?" he asked. "We've fooled around a bit, so I think we have chemistry, but he always pulls back and we end up cuddling. I thought it was cute, at first. We haven't talked about it, so I don't know if he wants to wait or what's holding him back exactly."

After we chatted through what was giving him so much anxiety about this situation, Carlo was able to organize his thoughts and decided to bring it up on their next date. Over dinner, Carlo opened up about how he was feeling about their lack of a sex life. "I really enjoy myself with you and it has felt so easy to be with you these past couple months. I feel that we haven't been able to explore our sexual connection as much as I would like to though. I'm a really sexual person and it seems like you aren't as interested in sex as I am. If that's true, I don't think this relationship is going to work. I don't want to pressure you; I just want to share how I've been feeling and why I've been acting a little weird lately."

His partner said that he understood, and that he was afraid sex was becoming an issue for them as well. He shared with Carlo that he had always had a hard time opening up sexually and hoped that if he found the right partner it would just happen naturally. He then became emotional, saying that this was the closest he had come to being in a relationship with someone and that he didn't feel any shift in his ability to be more physical with Carlo than he already had. He told Carlo, "I think this is a big block for me. I'm so sorry that you've been feeling this way, but I get it. I think I may need to talk to someone about the blocks I have around my sexuality. If I can't overcome them with you, someone who has been so great these past couple months, I think I really need to work on it on my own."

As hard as all of this was for both Carlo and his partner, the two of them ended the night feeling really close to one another and agreed that they would like to stay in each other's lives for as long as it made sense. "I wish things had gone differently, because he's so amazing," Carlo said in our session directly following the breakup. "It just wasn't meant to be. If anything, though, he showed me that I can take my time with new partners, but that without a strong sexual connection I can't go beyond being just friends."

How to Break Up Based on How Long You've Been Together: A Primer

Are you on the brink of a breakup but not sure what the proper code of conduct is? Here's a handy guide for communicating that you want to break up based on how long you've known someone and some sample language to do so. Keep in mind that this is just a guide. You can decide which mode of communication feels right given your unique relationship to the person.

- Zero to two months—text, phone, or in person
  › Sample language: "Hey, I've had a great time getting to know you. I just don't think we're a good match long term/I think we're looking for different things."
- Three to six months—phone, video call, or in person
  › Sample language: Identify what you like about the person and where there is a misalignment. "I think you're amazing, smart, and super sexy. I just know that I don't want kids and that's something you're

looking for. I truly want you to have that, but it just can't be with me."

- Six or more months—in person unless something terrible happened
  › Knowing someone longer may mean that you have to have several conversations over time about what's not working in the relationship. Whenever possible, use the SBI model to express how you're feeling and what you think about how the relationship is going.

*

BREAKUP PLANS

You're now equipped with some tools to use when you feel you're on the brink of a breakup. This is part of making the process a little kinder and gentler for everyone involved. Another part is creating a breakup plan that includes actions that can help support you and your partner as you move from coupledom to single units again. Just like you created a dating SOS plan, a breakup plan can help you be more intentional, as well as remind you of ways to care for yourself when things feel really hard post-breakup.

Think about how you would like to be broken up with. I know it's not a super fun exercise, but give yourself a minute to either remember a time someone broke up with you or envision it happening now. What would you like this person to do or say? Is there a certain phrase they'd use to reassure you? Now flip this. How would you like to break things off with someone in the future? How would you like them to feel when all is said and done, and how can your actions align with this outcome?

My client Luka created a breakup plan that she kept in mind when she felt that a relationship may have run its course or if someone wanted to end things with her. It wasn't always perfect, but she found that having an ideal scenario for how she wanted things to go was extremely helpful. Below is a sketch of what she came up with.

> If someone wants to break up with me, I will respect their decision. If I don't understand why, I will ask for clarification but will understand if I don't get an answer I like or the person isn't sure. I will remind myself that both people have to want to be together for things to work.

> If I have to break up with someone, I will try to be as transparent and caring as I can. I'd like to talk to them in person if possible, in a private and comfortable place. I'd prefer to not break up in my apartment because if things don't go well, or I'm feeling too overwhelmed, I want to be able to leave.

Self-care during a breakup is really important. Think about what activities you can do to comfort yourself. How do you like to de-stress? Can you make a plan to just let yourself express whatever you need to through journaling, crying, being creative, or whatever else helps you process? Here's Luka's post-breakup self-care ritual.

Before a potential breakup conversation, I may be too anxious to take care of myself by getting enough sleep or eating properly. I will remember to get as much sleep as I can afterward and even treat myself to a comforting meal. If I can, I will do yoga and take small walks each day to keep my body moving because I know even a little movement helps me stay grounded.

You don't have to go through a breakup alone. Who are the people you know you can turn to for support, who won't judge you for ending a relationship or being broken up with? Luka included her friend in her breakup plan as someone she could turn to when she needed support.

After a breakup, I will call my friend Sylvie to let her know how everything went. She's great at reminding me to rest and go easy on myself when I'm being too harsh. If possible, I'll schedule some time to hang out with her too. In addition, I will see my therapist regularly to check in and have space to process.

EXERCISE: CREATING YOUR OWN BREAKUP PLAN

Consider the following:

- How do I want to be broken up with? How do I want to break up with someone?
- What can I do to take care of myself after a breakup?

- Who can I turn to when I need support after a breakup?

The most experienced daters will tell you that breakups can be hard and emotionally draining. Even when you part ways amicably, there can still be a sense of loss and feelings of despair as you regroup and try to figure out what to do next. Figuring out whether you want to stay in or leave a relationship is tricky too! It's hard to know if you're experiencing a make-or-break moment or just panicking. Sometimes addressing how you're feeling can set the relationship back on course, or you might find that a split is imminent. We could all stand to be a bit kinder and gentler when it comes to ending relationships, so that's why creating a breakup plan can support you whether you're the one initiating a breakup or on the receiving end. It may feel like a bummer to make a plan to experience a breakup, but knowing how you can take care of yourself will help you heal a little easier when breakups happen.

13

You Survived! Now Thrive.

> If your knowledge were your wealth,
> then it would be well-earned.
>
> **—ERYKAH BADU**

After learning more about what you want and who you want it with, you found the kind of connection you were looking for, ditched the apps, and are feeling pretty good! So now what? The simple answer is to just enjoy yourself, but that's not as easy as it sounds. When faced with a promising new relationship or sexual partners, a tiny seed of doubt might appear. What if this all falls apart? What if we aren't as good for each other as we think we are? What happens next?! All of these are common questions that may or may not dissipate as you move into a steady rhythm with your partner. In fact, a little doubt, even when things are going really well, could be helpful for maintaining interest and keeping you from slipping into complacency. So if you feel a little unsteady even though you've "arrived," just know that it's not necessarily a bad thing, or a reason to throw in the towel.

The belief that once you've found what you're looking for things should be easy isn't entirely founded in reality. Of course, many folks find that when they're dating people they can be themselves with, the process of opening up and being vulnerable feels much easier than when this isn't the case. But that doesn't mean that these relationships are completely flawless.

Every relationship is relational. We are affected by each other's moods, desires, and stressors, as well as the things that bring the other joy. We have good days, bad days, and blah days when we just can't see past our immediate wants. All of this impacts how we are in a relationship with our partners and, believe it or not, it's what makes relationships with others so dynamic and enjoyable. Occasional friction allows us to learn more about each other and be better able to understand what the other person needs when the going gets tough.

We live in a time when many folks believe that most things in life can be optimized. For instance, if they drink a certain number of glasses of water a day, feed the body the right nutrients, and move regularly, they will function optimally. And that may work for a while for some people—until it doesn't. Because health is so much more than doing things optimally. It requires a holistic approach that examines everything, including one's environment, family history, community support, individual risk factors, and unique immunity.

Likewise, a relationship's health is not determined by the number of times you have sex or fight. And the goal isn't to always do things perfectly or prevent anything bad from ever happening. Holistically speaking, relationship health is measured by what happens when the people involved relate to one another over time and how that dynamic feels to each person. The factors that can impact relationship health are too many to name, but the big ones I see as a coach are communication, stress, and intimacy. While most people probably recognize the importance of these factors, the meaning they hold is usually quite different for each person. It is through the process of relating that people find common meaning—developing an understanding of how each person sees communication, stress, and intimacy differently.

We've covered the many ways in which communication plays a role in the early stages of relationships. General communication about who we are and what we want can take us far, and sexual communication can improve the quality of sex, but there's also communication about what we need from others, which can be really tricky to navigate. Without good communication about what each person needs, folks can start to feel alone even within a partnership.

In my practice, I talk a lot about the silent relationship and sex killer: stress. You might be aware of how stress impacts you, but what about how it affects your partner? And what do you do when, like so many of my clients who cohabitated during the pandemic, you're both trying to navigate stress in every aspect of life together? Even in the absence of a pandemic, the ways we handle stress (or not) impact the quality of our relationships.

Feeling intimately connected to a partner is a big indicator of relationship health. There is a signal-to-noise ratio of connection that ebbs and flows throughout the relationship's lifespan. We won't always feel totally connected with our partners; that's just life. But how couples are able to strengthen their signal of intimacy when they need to reconnect after the noise of life has interfered can really impact relationship health.

The degree to which each person in the relationship is willing to accept and work with each other's differences will also impact the health of the relationship. No two people will view all of life's problems the same way, and they won't come up with the exact same solutions. In fact, that's what makes relationships so beneficial. We need other people to help us see life in ways we couldn't otherwise envision.

There's so much to learn and do once you've found what you're looking for. But get excited! This is when the real fun begins. In this final chapter, we'll explore how to stay present for the next phase of connection: building relationships. You'll learn ways to be a better communicator, create more intimacy between you and your partner, and set some shared relationship goals so you can stop asking "What if?" and start planning your actual future together.

HOW TO BUILD DEEPER COMMUNICATION WITH YOUR PARTNER(S)

There are so many facets to communication, but the one that has been shown to have the biggest impact on general relationship satisfaction is how well we communicate our own needs and tend to each other's.* The expectations we have

---

* John M. Gottman and Joan DeClaire, *The Relationship Cure: A Five-Step Guide for Building Better Connections with Family, Friends, and Lovers* (New York: Crown, 2001), 1–26.

for how others will respond to our needs are largely dependent on how needs were met (or not) in our family of origin. Likewise, how we respond to the needs of others is built on entrenched patterns we may have adopted early in life and used consistently throughout all of our relationships. While we all have our own ways, one of the benefits of being in an intimate partnership is having someone who will turn toward us in our time of need. This can be both a comfort and a source of anxiety for many people who are newly partnered.

Most folks search high and low for people they can trust and be their full self with, but it can still feel scary to open up and communicate what they need in the relationship as things develop over time. When I work with couples as a sex coach, the number one thing we discuss is communication—how to communicate sexual needs and also general needs within the relationship. Like many folks, my clients often believe that since they found the "right" people, they shouldn't have to explain themselves. The other person should intuitively understand all of their wants and needs. Never mind the fact that they know deep down that they don't have the ability to do the same for their partner. I don't blame anyone for having this belief, though. I blame the widespread cultural expectation that partnership means "you complete me."

The idea that, somehow, someway, another person will be able to anticipate what you need from moment to moment and fill every void because of a supernatural bond is far-fetched and, frankly, unhelpful. The result of this type of thinking is a stonewall effect in the relationship, where one partner is awaiting instruction while the other sits in silence expecting them to be equipped with this knowledge already.

Recognizing this tendency to assume that someone has all the information they need about you already filed away when you meet them is the first step in breaking the stonewalling cycle.

That's exactly what caused a breakthrough for my clients Tim and Samara, who knew that they needed better communication skills and had already done a lot in other areas of their relationship to strengthen their connection. But when it came down to regularly sharing their wants and needs within the relationship, there was hesitation on both sides. To start, they both thought that their bond was enough to get them through any rough patches without having to explain much, which was true to a degree. But when problems did arise, it took so long to get to a place of understanding that, by the time they had reached a détente, they were left with a trail of hurt feelings to patch up.

Some of the discord stemmed from the communication assumption they had for each other. They each assumed that the other would raise any concerns they had about the relationship, so a lack of tough conversations and arguments had lulled them both into a false sense of security. While sex was the main focus of our discussions, this assumption persisted throughout the relationship. This is actually pretty common—we all would like to believe that the people we care about most will feel comfortable bringing their concerns to our attention. The problem is that this assumption doesn't take into account how difficult it is to actually talk to a partner about what's bothering you, whether or not it has to do with them. A lot of folks find it much easier to stuff down feelings of frustration than to discuss them openly. This is why arguments about something small, like someone leaving a sock on the bedroom floor, can erupt into something way bigger. Eventually, those stuffed frustrations spill over.

Tim and Samara were in a stalemate about sex because what wasn't being said was that he needed sex more frequently and casually, and she needed to feel more excited by the sex they were having. As it stood, she wasn't into the kind of sex that was on offer. Every couple of months, they would have a huge fight that left them both feeling dejected and depleted. Their pattern was to not talk about the everyday concerns they each had—some related to sex and some not— and over time these stuffed frustrations would be too much to tamp down. It wasn't that Samara didn't have her own desires almost as regularly as Tim; it was that she couldn't quite understand why sex always felt rushed and not focused on her pleasure. Over the course of their relationship, she'd refused Tim's requests for sex so many times (even when she was feeling her own desire for it) that he had given up on asking. She never felt comfortable initiating sex, so this left them both with independent sex lives. When they came to work with me, they shared that they both had a regular masturbation practice but that it had been months since they'd experienced sex together. This arrangement might work for some, but it was a far cry from what Tim and Samara had envisioned for themselves when they had gotten together two years ago. They wanted to figure out what was blocking their sexual connection and get back to feeling closer to each other in the relationship.

So we started small. They both had to practice communicating their needs in low-stakes, nonsexual situations. Where they had been resistant or even fearful to verbalize what they needed, they were encouraged to try, see what happened, and track their results. From asking for a hug and a cup of tea when she was upset by a work issue to requesting some alone time over the weekend when he felt a little suffocated after working from home all week together, they both got more comfortable airing their needs rather than stuffing them. And what really got them talking was how, when they communicated a need, the other person was great at meeting that need if they could.

It took some time for both Tim and Samara to pinpoint what they needed and even more time to get comfortable with verbalizing this to one another. But in the end this is what helped them bridge their sexual gap. As we covered earlier when we discussed sexual feedback, part of being able to communicate your needs is recognizing what they are, and that can be difficult. Additionally, what we need changes, and it's sometimes hard to pin down our general mood or the emotions we feel as things get stirred up for seemingly no reason. Remember the basic emotions we covered in Chapter 7 when we discussed vulnerability? As a refresher, they are fear, anger, sadness, joy, disgust, surprise, trust, and anticipation. If you have a hard time recognizing what you feel, you can use these as a way to take your emotional temperature. Then, if you think there are any other related feelings, you can add those in. Sometimes just saying "I'm angry" can be really helpful, especially if your partner is completely in the dark about what's going on with you.

After recognizing how you feel, the next step is communicating what you need. Over time, Tim was able to share that when he felt really happy with Samara, it was a turn-on. He wanted to show her through his actions how he was feeling toward her. She could see his perspective but countered with how intense his desire for sex felt for her. She told him that, rather than a display of his affection, it felt like a demand for sexual gratification. This led them into a series of conversations about how they could get their sexual needs met in a way that felt amazing for both of them. Samara needed Tim to consider *when* he was making his advances. She reflected back to him that often he tried initiating sex when she was in the middle of a stressful day or at night when she was really tired. This timing made sex feel more like a chore or an annoyance. He could see this as a barrier to her wanting to have sex with him.

In our work together, we focused on what makes sex great for both of them and tried to find middle ground. Tim became better at choosing his moments, and if it wasn't right for Samara, she expressed why and proposed an alternative time they could both look forward to. Samara even became more comfortable initiating sex when she wanted to because she was feeling less pressure to be sexual when she wasn't ready. It also helped that they were able to have sex that focused more on the things she enjoyed, like oral sex and a little role play. She shared that this was a huge incentive for her to want to have sex and ask for it.

HOW MUCH IS TOO MUCH?

While communicating one's needs in a relationship is super important, it has its limits. A common relationship communication pattern that can cause unnecessary problems is actually the flip side of withholding and stonewalling and involves being overly critical and talking everything to death. Remember that relationships are relational, so it's not just how you perceive the other person's behaviors and how they affect you that counts. Your partner's intentions might be very different from the impact that their behaviors have, so you have to take time to get to the root. We all misspeak or make careless mistakes, and relationships are about figuring out how to understand the other person, flaws and all. Hopefully, your partner is doing the same thing with you!

Recognizing what you like and don't like about your partner is great, and it's good to have a grasp of when what they do impacts you, but it's also a good idea to check in with yourself about whether the behavior and your response to it warrant a full conversation. Sometimes other people are annoying, even the ones we care deeply for. That doesn't mean we have to tell them every time they do something that annoys us. This overcommunication can cause excessive friction in the relationship, making it hard for one, or both, of you to relax and be yourselves. This can be a huge barrier to intimacy.

Being critical and overly communicative about the things that rub you the wrong way is actually an extension of that unhelpful "you complete me" belief. If this person is your match, then they should be perfect, right? They should fit into your life without question or pushback. And if they do anything that displeases you, that calls into question the whole relationship. In some cases, how we feel about our partner's behavior is a very good indicator of whether they're a good match. But other times, it's simply faultfinding and can make your partner feel really bad about themselves.

If you know that you have a tendency toward faultfinding, think about creating your own mental scale for determining when to bring things up. For instance, the low end of the scale is "annoying" and the high end is "insulting" or "disrespectful." Think about where the action falls on the scale and, if it skews low and everything else is going great, consider skipping the feedback. The only exception to this rule would be if there's a particular behavior that happens frequently. Frequency is definitely a factor that can swing an annoying behavior over to the disrespectful side of the scale, especially if you bring it to the other person's attention and they continue to do it.

While some degree of annoyance is expected in any relationship occasionally, the general goal is to develop habits of communication that allow you both to acknowledge your differences and move on. Some people are more difficult to be around when they are emotionally upset or stressed out, and all relationships go through bad patches, but prolonged periods of bad or toxic communication may point to larger concerns. You don't have to stand idly by when things get rough. Sometimes you will need outside support for your relationship, and sometimes even that won't be enough to keep the relationship going.

RELATIONSHIP CHECK-INS

So many relationships suffer because of poor communication and the resulting inability to meet each other's needs.

When needs aren't being met by the relationship, many people feel a lack of intimacy—that feeling of closeness we develop with partners over time. My clients often work through these issues generally with couples counseling and specifically through sex coaching with me, but they also use other tools to help improve intimacy. For instance, many of my clients allocate time in their week for checking in with each other. This is usually a semi-structured conversation that happens at regular intervals and can help provide a space to air things out as well as connect more deeply with what's going on in each other's lives. I have seen this work well for new couples and for those who have been together a long time and have lost track of each other in the day-to-day shuffle. During COVID, couples struggled with the realization that spending more time with each other didn't necessarily translate to more intimacy. In fact, this forced exposure to every little thing they did during the day made it harder to connect in meaningful ways.

I recommend relationship check-ins to anyone who feels like they talk to their partner about everything except the important stuff in life. I also recommend them to folks who feel more like "friends" or "roommates" than sexual or romantic partners. Relationship check-ins can be a standing thirty-minute conversation or a date night each week, or a state-of-the-union debrief once a month. Whatever the timing, be sure to include big, open-ended questions that can guide the conversation. These can be the same each time you check in. In fact, this consistency could help with making it more of a relationship ritual than a "meeting." Below are some sample questions you can use, but feel free to come up with ones that feel meaningful to you.

- What were the highlights of your week?
- What did you struggle most with this week?
- What are you looking forward to next week?
- What are you dreading next week?
- Is there anything you need from me to support you?

Take turns asking the questions and really listen to each other's responses. The questions above are helpful for getting to the core of what you and your partner are going through. Follow-up questions are great for getting clarity, especially about what you can do to support them. Sometimes whether someone feels supported is dependent upon how the support is given. Encourage each other to be as open and specific as possible. This will help both of you understand each other better.

You can regularly schedule these check-ins with your partner or use them on an as-needed basis. You can always increase or decrease the frequency depending on how you're both feeling. Sometimes you may not feel the need for check-ins at all, and other times they can be really helpful to have more often. The main point is that you give yourselves the time and the space to express what's going on and remain open to the other person's joys and concerns.

SETTING SHARED RELATIONSHIP GOALS AND EXPECTATIONS

It may feel like it's too soon to start planning a future with a new partner, but there is a benefit to having a little foresight and something to work toward together. First and foremost, this can give you both a framework to use as you're deepening your relationship. For instance, exploring whether or not to eventually cohabitate is a great way to understand where each person sees the relationship heading. You might find it helpful to know that you both feel like cohabitation is a goal you would like to move toward. And if one of you wants to cohabitate and the other wholly objects to this idea, there may be other goals you can focus on, like traveling together or just generally spending more time together. Another goal might be to keep things casual and communicate with each other if that arrangement isn't working for one person or the other.

A second reason why shared goals in relationships are helpful is that they can manage expectations. Take the example of a couple in which cohabitation isn't an option for one of them. Knowing that up front and then deciding together where they'd like to take the relationship can be really helpful for keeping both parties grounded in what the relationship dynamic is, rather than individually trying to guess at what happens next. That's when misalignments can happen—one person believes that the relationship is moving in one direction and the other person is on another track completely. The result can be disappointment on both sides.

Creating shared relationship goals can be a very organic process or something that is explicitly stated. The more you learn about each other's needs and what you each want your future to look like, the more you can both start to shape a shared vision for how you fit in each other's worlds. Shared goals and expectations can keep everyone on the same track, whether that's agreeing to see each other casually or focus on the long term. And, like everything else in life, what those goals are might shift and change over time.

That was the case for my client Isabella, who had been seeing her partner for about nine months. When they first met, they both wanted to keep things casual. Isabella was putting herself through grad school and working long hours, so she didn't have much time to give to someone else. She expressed this early on and was met with enthusiasm from her partner, who had been seeing a few other people at that time. They had a shared goal of enjoying their time together when they could, without putting too much pressure on each other to hang out, and that's exactly what they did. And then, one night when they were on a date, they realized that they had been happily seeing each other a couple times a week for the past two months. Isabella had graduated, freeing her time up tremendously, and her partner wasn't dating anyone else anymore. Could it be time to revise the goal?

Isabella shared that she was conflicted about committing more to her partner. While she really cared for them and had developed a strong connection, she worried that she might ruin what they had by asking for more.

"We agreed that this arrangement worked for both of us and to keep things light. What if they still want that?" she asked.

I encouraged her to share how she was feeling and see how they responded. "You both are in very different places than when you first met. You've managed to stay in each other's lives for this long, so even if they aren't interested in more I think you'll both figure out how to shift your relationship. Maybe you get a long-term partner out of this, or maybe a really good friend. The hardest part will be telling them how you feel."

One night over drinks, Isabella brought up the fact that she was reconsidering their shared goal of keeping things casual. "I think I need more, and I can see a future together where we're more committed. Is that something you'd be interested in trying?"

Much to her excitement, her partner said that they had been thinking the same thing. "I haven't enjoyed myself with anyone as much as I've enjoyed my time with you. I think we should try and see what happens!"

Isabella was ecstatic when we discussed how the conversation went. She had never felt a relationship evolve as easily as it had with her partner, and she felt that was a really good sign for things to come.

Some of my clients have major life goals that they agree to quite early on with new partners. Like Tessa, who had been dating for years to find someone to start a family with. The search had been long and hard, but she found someone she connected with values-wise. As a father of a small child, he was also open to expanding his family with the right person. About a year after working with me, she wrote to tell me that they were talking about having a baby.

Another client, Lissane, worked with me to find kink partners. One of her relationship goals with one of her partners was to explore her dominant side. Her partner was also new to kink and the two of them were a good chemistry match. Lissane wasn't 100 percent confident that she wanted an exclusively dominant-submissive relationship, but she wanted to give herself the opportunity to learn more about what appealed to her about domination. Her partner helped her create space to try things out, and in the end they both learned more about what they were looking for. When her partner decided to pursue someone else whose specific dom style appealed more to him, she acquiesced, knowing that they had actually achieved the goals they wanted to work on together.

Being open to how goals unfold is one of the ways my clients get the most from their relationship experiences. Whether those relationships are short-lived or long-term, when each person is invested in moving the relationship toward these goals, that's when all the hard work of dating really pays off. It's when everyone gets to reap the reward of finding people who want not only to understand them but also to build with them, and the power of that cannot be overstated.

EXERCISE: REFLECTING ON YOUR PROGRESS

Your final exercise is to take a few minutes to reflect on how far you've come. Whether you've recently updated your dating profile or settled into a routine with a new partner, what are the wins you can celebrate right now? Use the below prompts to help you.

If you're still searching:

How has your perspective on dating and how you want to date changed? What are you doing differently that feels really good?

If you are partnered:

How does this new person (or these new people) align with your values? How does the connection you found support you being your most authentic self?

It is my hope that you have found relationships that truly work for you, and if not, that you at least feel like you're on your way. I also hope that you have started to think about relationships more as opportunities for growth and learning than as successes and failures. Each person you invite into your life will lead you further down the path of your own self-discovery, which is ultimately what we are all here to do for each other. Along the way, you will get to experience all of your partners' weird quirks, the joy they bring to your life, and how they see the world. By relating to who they are, you get to share the greatest, most fun aspect of humanity: connection.

Conclusion

Dating can sometimes feel like you're embarking on a long, arduous journey on your own, or that there's something that everyone else but you just seems to "get." After reading this book, you should have a greater appreciation for the fact that every single person is trying to figure out the dating world so they can find what they want. And just like you, they are experiencing the peaks and valleys of putting their unique desires on display for the world to see so they can find connections that work for them.

When folks whose desires align finally get together, it can be truly amazing! But if you get bogged down in the "right way" to date, you can miss out on matches who could not only meet but exceed your desires. Too often we overlook people who have a lot to offer us as partners in the short or long term because of ideas about dating we inherited, instead of relying on our own internal guides about what's best for us. My greatest hope is that this book has broken down some walls and dispelled some myths that keep folks from experiencing all the joys that dating can provide.

You did a lot of work throughout this book, starting with unpacking some unhelpful ideas you had about what dating should be. Whether that was letting go of a timeline for finding your person that was based on your family's expectations, or saying no to rigid ideas you had about what makes a person good enough to date, or even releasing negative scripts about your own worthiness to have the kind of sex you really want. Centering yourself and what makes you happy is the only way you can begin to truly find what you're looking for.

This book is meant as a framework for moving through the dating process while keeping the bigger picture in mind. It's not easy staying the course sometimes, and if you're not careful you can burn out before you even get to have a little fun. Sometimes you put in all the work to find a dating app that meets your needs, carefully vet your matches, and set up dates—only to be ghosted, catfished, or breadcrumbed. It's no wonder some folks want no part of dating these days! But you now have your own goals for dating; you've named them and maybe even accomplished one or two while reading this book. You have tools for sticking with the process, like red and green flags and a dating schedule that keeps you focused without becoming overwhelmed. You've also set yourself up to have dates you'll enjoy no matter what, and you created ways to reject people kindly when it's time to move on. You know that ghosting and breadcrumbing are just ways people show you that they're not ready for what you have to give.

And you know that there are plenty of other folks out there who will be.

You've looked back on your past dating experience with more kindness toward yourself and others, because you now know that you were just trying to figure out what you wanted back then and so were your partners. We don't always get it perfectly right in dating, but that doesn't mean we can't keep trying and learning and refining until we get something that feels fun and exciting. You also know that showing empathy toward others while dating is a great way to give folks a real chance. Each person we meet has their own story, and sometimes just being available for connection, regardless of the outcome, is what can make the process of dating more joyful. Dating is one of the ways we get to share our stories with each other in the interest of seeing what's really there. Sometimes what's there is a night of pleasant conversation, and other times it's the start of something meaningful for both of you.

In each chapter, I highlighted what a big part sexuality plays in dating, whether you want to hook up or not. Now that you know all of your sexual values, you can use them to assess how compatible you are with folks before you even have sex. You should feel more confident identifying what you want sexually and know that you have the tools to give sexual feedback when necessary. This is often where dating journeys can go off course, but knowing how to express your wants can get you back on track and into some pretty mind-blowing sexual territory. Maybe you've already experienced this. Trust me, there's more of that to come (pun intended) as you practice the very important skill of giving and receiving sexual feedback.

Every single person deserves the right to find the best sex and dating experiences for them. The upsetting truth is that dating is harder for some people than others. There's way more to dating than just showing up and being your best, because often the best you is, for any number of reasons, undesirable to other people. People of color, women, femmes, and nonbinary and LGBTQIA+ folks deserve to feel safe and seen while dating, and this isn't always the case. Fat folks will suffer the indignities of being overlooked based on fatphobia and anti-fat bias. Those with disabilities and mental-health concerns will struggle amid dating apps' incredibly restrictive and homogenous cultural expectations of desirability.

We need to acknowledge the unequal playing field in dating, because it is real. And we need to use the access that online dating gives us to connect with people who will actually support us and recognize our unique goals and desires. There are a lot of things we can't control in dating, but, with a better understanding of what they are, we can get through them to the things that we can control, like who we share ourselves and our time with. All of the isms on dating apps can make the journey fraught with anxiety and pain for some daters. It can be difficult to find the fun in a process that bases so much on how we look. We can't escape how people read us; all we can do is be who we are and trust that there are people out there who will value that. This requires a vulnerability that lots of folks find hard to muster. And I get that! Dating as a minority is no small feat. But my personal experience and the experiences of my clients have shown me that this type of vulnerability pays off in major ways, including sex with people who are all about you, relationships built on an honest assessment of shared values and goals, and a growing sense of self-love for being unapologetically who you are.

The truths of who you are and what you want are your greatest assets in dating. You can vet your matches extensively before meeting them in person. You can ask them the hard questions about what they believe and stand for, and you can tell folks to educate themselves on the matters that are close to your heart. You don't have to apologize for wanting whatever you want in the way that you want it. Many folks have never had to apologize for these things, so why should you?

Finding people with whom we can truly connect and the experiences we get to share with them are the rewards of dating, and we only reap those rewards if we are open to them. Some of us will get small glimpses of this, while others get to revel in the fun of the game that dating has become. However frequently or infrequently we get to experience these joys, it's important to acknowledge how great it is to ask for exactly what you want and receive it. If folks are swiping and matching and dating and sexing with more intention, the world will be a better, safer, and more fun place to date.

Because the connections we make in dating can sometimes be fleeting, it's also important to recognize the value of breakups. They can be painful, yes, but they can also be opportunities to take a step back and assess how you can get more of the good stuff from your next experience—whether that's taking the lessons you learned about your sexuality with one partner and carrying those into new sexual relationships or recognizing fundamental values differences that you know you need to avoid for deeper partnerships in the future.

And in those amazing moments when you're in awe of what you've found because you stayed open but also aware of your own goals and firm in your truths, you can settle into enjoying where your journey has led you. There is so much to explore beyond the often narrow views we have about sex and relationships. Rather than being about getting the best, I want more people to see a world of possibility when it comes to connection. I hope you, like my clients, have unlocked in yourself the belief that dating doesn't have to be a painful chore until it just magically makes sense somehow. It's *your* dating life, and it's supposed to be fun.

Acknowledgments

This book is dedicated to the memory of my uncle, David Edwards. As the first openly gay person in my life, he showed me what living one's truth meant and had a lot of fun in the process.

Boundless gratitude goes to Geoff Vasile for celebrating all my wins with me and helping me through the hard stuff, including taking care of me when I had COVID and a deadline to make. For my mom, I am so appreciative of our relationship and the encouragement you've given me my entire life. I know I'm not perfect, but I'm so grateful to have a mom in whose eyes I am, no matter what.

A shout-out to my besties, who have supported me through thick and thin and know exactly what I mean when I say that. Thank you Carolyn for the rad brainstorming sessions that produced the title of this book. Thank you Jenn, Leah, Melissa, and Sharon for your love and encouragement.

Thank you Angie for being a constant friend and food companion. Thanks to Dania for proofreading my book proposal and for grounding chats and walks. Thank you Ann, George, Michael, and Nancy Jo for your words of encouragement as I endeavored to follow in your footsteps as published authors.

To all of my loving and supportive family, thank you for accepting me as a sex coach. It is not lost on me how cool that is! Lots of gratitude to the Mariage family for letting me write in their cottage and Tom and Sara Edwards for helping me navigate all the fine print.

Thank you Maggie Auffarth and Erin Niumata of Folio Literary Management for helping me bring a dream to life. Big thanks to the folks at Seal Press, especially Emi Ikkanda for believing in the book and Kyle Gipson for your amazing editing support. Thanks to Rebecca McCusker and Amie Byrd of Creative Content Shop. It has been so valuable to have your thoughts and support along the way.

I would like to acknowledge the many teachers I've had, mainly women, who shaped my worldview and helped me develop my voice. To Dr. Patti Britton, I thank you for not only training me as a sex coach, but also showing me how valuable what we do is.

Finally, thank you to my clients, workshop participants, and students over the years for providing inspiration for the book and showing me that there was a need for it to exist.

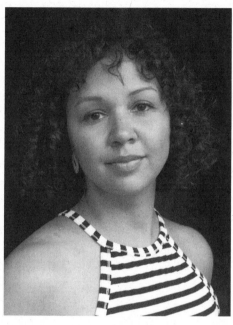

HELENA PRICE

Myisha Battle is a certified clinical sexologist and sex and dating coach, educator, and speaker. She holds a master's in psychology from The New School for Social Research. Her expertise has been featured in the *Washington Post*, *New York Magazine*'s *The Cut*, *Refinery29*, *Oprah Magazine*, *San Francisco Chronicle*, *Playboy*, and *Nylon*, among many others. She lives in San Francisco, California.